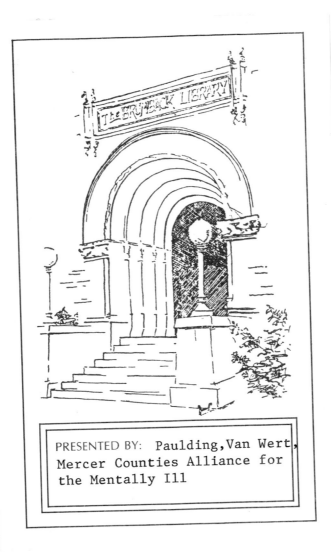

THE BRUMBACK LIBRARY

ADVANCE PRAISE

"For over twenty-five years, Rosalynn Carter has been educating America about mental illness. Her efforts to destigmatize the issue and advocate for those affected are nothing short of extraordinary. Her sensitive book is an invaluable guide to all whose lives are touched by mental illness."　　—BETTY FORD

"With her new book, Mrs. Carter not only recognizes the impact this disease has on individuals, but also the toll it can take on family and friends. This insightful guide is a valuable resource for anyone whose life has been affected by mental illness."

—TIPPER GORE, mental health policy advisor to the President

"With this compassionate and singularly helpful book, Rosalynn Carter continues her impressive public service commitment to the mentally ill. It should prove extremely useful to family members, patients, and community professionals."　　—KAY REDFIELD JAMISON, professor of psychiatry,
Johns Hopkins School of Medicine,
and author of *An Unquiet Mind*

"An important resource for families, friends, and those facing the challenges of mental illness. It delivers its message with warmth, clarity, and candor."

—LAURIE FLYNN, executive director,
National Alliance for the Mentally Ill.

"Rosalynn Carter—no surprise—has done her homework, and has put together a thorough, compassionate, specific, and eminently useful handbook for those who themselves suffer from mental illness and especially for families and friends who must deal with the fallout and the stigma."　　—MIKE WALLACE

"Family and friends will want to turn to Mrs. Carter's book first for empathy, information, and advice."　　—C. EVERETT KOOP, M.D.

"Mrs. Carter's book offers an amazing amount of good information and a clear, compassionate perspective of mental health issues and the needs of individuals and families touched by mental illnesses."

—MICHAEL M. FAENZA, M.S.S.W., president and CEO,
National Mental Health Association

"A compassionate, very valuable book. Rosalynn Carter reminds us why she was, and is, such a beloved first lady."　　—JOANNE WOODWARD

"Rosalynn Carter has given us an extraordinary book, invaluable to those whose families and friends are touched by mental illness. She gives reason for hope and also wonderful guidance on compassionate, sensitive caring."

—HERB PARDES, M.D., dean of the faculty of medicine,
Columbia University College of Physicians and Surgeons

"You're walking out of the doctor's office, stunned. What, a member of my family has mental illness? Where do I turn first? Let me recommend Mrs. Carter's book as a great comfort and source of information."
—TONY RANDALL

"Mrs. Carter says what needs to be said: That mental illnesses are real, that they can be diagnosed, and that effective treatments exist. This is a book that will inform and offer hope to individuals and families who today are grappling with the still grim realities of disabling mental disorders."
—STEVEN E. HYMAN, M.D., director,
National Institute of Mental Health

"This book will demystify mental illness for those of us who suffer from it and for those who suffer because of us. I have no doubt it's going to help erase so much of the stigma attached to what is seen by so many people as either a character weakness or something evil. I especially appreciate the emphasis on prevention and management of mental illness through awareness and vigilance."
—MARGOT KIDDER

"This book is a prescription for action—a blueprint for transforming ignorance to knowledge, passivity to power, and most important, despair to hope."
—MARTHA M. MANNING, Ph.D., author of
Undercurrents: A Life Beneath the Surface

"A book like this is most important for a truly compassionate and enlightening picture of the pain and suffering of mental illnesses. It also offers the definite possibility of hope. Mrs. Carter should be saluted for her passionate dedication."
—ROD STEIGER

"A very informative book that puts a human face on a much-misunderstood problem. It will help those who suffer and their families who love them."
—ALMA POWELL

"This is a remarkable account by the foremost advocate for improving our understanding of mental health and mental illness. Mrs. Carter shows us lucidly how this understanding will lead to improved care of those who are ill and how to combat the stigma long associated with mental illness. This book should be widely read to move us toward a more informed, compassionate society."
—JULIUS B. RICHMOND, M.D., professor of health policy,
Department of Social Medicine, Harvard Medical School,
and former assistant secretary of health and Surgeon General,
and first director of the National Head Start Program

Also by Rosalynn Carter

First Lady from Plains

Everything to Gain: Making the Most of the Rest of Your Life
(with Jimmy Carter)

Helping Yourself Help Others: A Book for Caregivers
(with Susan K. Golant)

Helping Someone with Mental Illness

Helping Someone with Mental Illness

A Compassionate Guide
for Family, Friends, and Caregivers

Rosalynn Carter

with Susan K. Golant

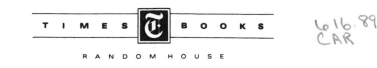

TIMES BOOKS

RANDOM HOUSE

The identities of all individuals to whom we have referred by first name only in this book have been disguised in name and physical description to protect their privacy.

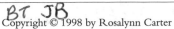
Grateful acknowledgment is made to the following for permission to reprint previously published material:

The Journal for the California Alliance for the Mentally Ill: Excerpts from "Awakenings—to What?"
from the July 1996 issue (Volume 7, #2) of *The Journal for the California Alliance for the Mentally
Ill,* Dan E. Weisburd, Editor and Publisher. Copyright © 1996. Complete copies of this issue
may be obtained for $10 by writing to: The JOURNAL, 1111 Howe Avenue, Suite 475,
Sacramento, CA 95825. Reprinted by permission.

Alfred A. Knopf, Inc., and International Creative Management: Excerpts from *An Unquiet Mind*
by Kay Redfield Jamison. Copyright © 1995 by Kay Redfield Jamison. Rights in the British
Commonwealth are controlled by International Creative Management. Reprinted
by permission of Alfred A. Knopf, Inc., and International Creative Management.

The New York Times: Excerpt from an Op-Ed article by A. M. Rosenthal from November 23,
1990. Copyright © 1990 by The New York Times Company. Reprinted by permission.

Sigma Theta Tau International: Close paraphrasing and summarization of "The Caregiver Career"
from *IMAGE: The Journal of Nursing Scholarship* (Issue 25, 1993, p. 214). Reprinted
by permission of Sigma Theta Tau International.

Times Books, a division of Random House, Inc.: Excerpts from *Today's Children* by David Hamburg. Copyright © 1992 by David Hamburg. Reprinted by permission of Times Books,
a division of Random House, Inc.

Warner Bros. Publications U.S. Inc.: Excerpts from "Because You Loved Me" by Diane Warren
(with one-word lyric change: "baby" to "caregivers"). Copyright © 1996 by Realsongs
(ASCAP) and Touchstone Pictures Songs & Music, Inc. (ASCAP). All rights reserved. Used by
permission of Warner Bros. Publications U.S., Inc., Miami, FL 33014.

Library of Congress Cataloging-in-Publication Data
Carter, Rosalynn.
Helping someone with a mental illness: a compassionate guide for families, friends,
and caregivers / Rosalynn Carter, with Susan K. Golant.
p.   cm.
Includes bibliographical references and index.
ISBN 0-8129-2899-7 (alk. paper)
1. Mental illness—Popular works.   2. Consumer education.
I. Golant, Susan K.   II. Title.
RC454.4.C373   1998
616.89—dc21   97-39218

Random House website address: www.randomhouse.com
Printed in the United States of America

9   8   7   6   5   4   3   2
First Edition
Book design by Susan Hood

To all those who have taught me, guided me, and worked with me since I became involved with mental health issues.

Acknowledgments

This is a book I have wanted to write for a long time. So much progress has been made in the mental health field just in the last decade. With our new knowledge of the brain, medications and treatment methods for mental illnesses have changed dramatically. These illnesses can now be diagnosed, they can be treated, and the overwhelming majority of people who suffer can lead normal lives—living at home, working, being productive citizens. I want everyone to know that. I want them to know that most mental illnesses are biologically based, and that there should be no reason for shame or embarrassment if they or a member of their family is mentally ill, and that there is no need to suffer unnecessarily when help is available.

This book would not have been possible without the help of many people who have taught me, guided me, and worked with me since I became involved in the mental health field. I want to thank them and express my gratitude for their assistance and support over the years.

I am grateful to the staff of The Carter Center mental health program and our task force for their daily help and for the inspiration for this book. I am especially indebted to John Gates,

Ph.D., the director of the program, who read the manuscript as it was taking shape and offered many helpful suggestions.

Particular thanks go also to Kathy Cade with whom I have worked for years on mental health issues. She carefully reviewed the book and gave me detailed comments and advice that were of great assistance.

I want to thank my friends at the National Institute of Mental Health, especially Steve Hyman, M.D., for reviewing the chapters on research and providing comments to assure the accuracy of the information. Rex Cowdry, M.D., David Pickar, M.D., Susan Swedo, M.D., David Shore, M.D., Grayson Norquist, M.D., Stan Schneider, Ph.D., Richard Nakamura, Ph.D., Steve Moldin, Ph.D., and Marsha Corbett made valuable contributions. The NIMH also provided the illustrations of the brain.

There are many others who were of great assistance and to whom I owe a debt of gratitude: Claire Griffin-Francell, Kathy Cronkite, Rod Steiger, Don Richardson, Kenya Napper Bello, Terrence Caster, Beverly Long, Susan Daves, Jerilyn Ross, L.I.C.S.W., Stuart Perry, Larry Fricks, Judith Johnson, Angela Koppenol, Braxton Mallard, Jeffrey M. Schwartz, M.D., Victor Angeles, and Melbernita Herndon, all made important contributions. I am particularly grateful to those who let me tell their stories, some included above and many others whose names I have changed to protect their identity. These are courageous individuals, willing to share their own experiences in an effort to better the lives of others who suffer from mental illnesses.

I am also indebted to Madeline Edwards and Crystal Williams in our office in Plains, Lyn Nesbit, our longtime agent, and Betsy Rapoport, my editor, and her associates at Random House. Betsy encouraged me and guided me in making the book a very personal one.

It is difficult for me to express the gratitude, admiration and respect I feel for my coauthor, Susan Golant. I am fortunate to have the benefit of her ability to plan and organize the book as well as her knowledge of the subject. Writing this book took much research and study, more I think than either Susan or I anticipated when we first began the work. Without her help with both the research and writing, the book would not have been possible. I am grateful to her. I also want to express my thanks to Mitch Golant, Ph.D., Susan's husband, who made many helpful suggestions.

Finally, I want to thank my husband, Jimmy, for his love and patience over the many months that it has taken me to complete this book. He has edited my writings, helped me as I struggled to make the technical information about the brain and the various mental illnesses readable and understandable, and supported and encouraged me in every way.

—Rosalynn Carter

It has been both a privilege and an honor to work with Rosalynn Carter on this book. I am deeply indebted to her for her vision, integrity, and compassion and am grateful that she continues to place her trust in me. Her and President Carter's gracious and unwavering efforts to help those who are suffering will always serve as models to me.

I would also like to thank my agent, Robert E. Tabian, and our editor at Times Books, Betsy Rapoport, for their steadfast guidance and support. My soul mate and husband, Dr. Mitch Golant, has inspired me with his constant love and his will to "do good in the world"; our daughters Cherie and Aimee have given me a deep appreciation for the miracle of life; and my parents, Holocaust survivors, Arthur and Mary Kleinhandler, have demonstrated by extraordinary example the human capacity to heal. I am grateful to them all.

—Susan K. Golant, M.A.

Contents

Contents

Part I

The Legacy of Stigma

"Superman Will Die . . . Killed by a Superlunatic, an Escapee from a Cosmic Insane Asylum!" This was the headline in papers around the country heralding the Man of Steel's imminent death in a comic book released in September 1992. And just one month later, the newspapers in Georgia heralded "Six Flags over Georgia to Open New Halloween Attraction: Asylum of Horrors."

Those were the opening lines of a speech I gave in 1992. Unfortunately, media depictions that discriminate against those who suffer from mental illnesses and contribute to the stigma continue today.

"TV Ad Features Straitjacketed Man Ranting in Padded Cell." This headline was the subject of a Stigma Alert from the National Stigma Clearinghouse circulated to the mental health community in October 1997. The ad, jointly sponsored by

Universal Studios and Pepsi-Cola, aired throughout southern California, publicizing the Universal theme park's "Halloween Horror Nights." It showed a man wearing a straitjacket in a padded room, ranting and bouncing off the walls. A guard outside the cell was drinking a Pepsi-Cola. Exasperated, the guard shuts the peep door on the thirsty man inside.

Just a few months earlier, Nickelodeon released *Good Burger,* a summer movie for children, in which a subplot takes place in an asylum. The film's heroes are kidnapped, carted off in straitjackets, and thrown into a padded cell at "Demented Hills Asylum."

And when the bombing took place in Atlanta during the 1996 Summer Olympics, the headline of the local newspaper heralded, "Search Is on for 'Random Nut Case.'" And the article began, "The hunt for the Centennial Olympic Park bomber is likely to focus initially on home-grown terrorists or what police officials and security experts refer to as a 'random nut case.'"

❧

It seems as though I and many others have been fighting myths, misconceptions, and stereotypes about mental illnesses for decades. And although much has changed over the years, we can see from the media coverage that much is left to be done. Why else would *60 Minutes* veteran Mike Wallace admit about his own depression, "I just didn't want people to know of my vulnerability. I was ashamed. It was a confession of weakness. For years, depression meant the crazy house."[1]

And why else would actress Margot Kidder, following a much publicized episode of mental illness, confess that she'd rather be thought of as an alcoholic and drug abuser than a person with manic-depression? As she told Barbara Walters in a televised interview, "Mental illness is the last taboo. It's the one that scares everyone to death, and I have to include myself in that until the last few months."

Would either of these famous people have felt the same had they been diagnosed with a physical illness such as diabetes or high blood pressure? Despite the growing body of knowledge, a tremendous gap still exists between what the experts know about brain-related illnesses and what the public understands. The challenges involved in promoting better mental health for all Americans are many and complex, but none demands more of our attention than that of society's attitudes toward mentally ill individuals.

It didn't take long for me to learn about the impact of stigma when I first began working in the field. I would call mental health meetings when Jimmy was governor of Georgia, and the only people to show up would be a handful of dedicated advocates and a few government employees, who probably came only because my husband was governor. At that time, no one would admit to having a mental illness; no one would acknowledge that a family member was suffering. Funding for mental health programs was always inadequate. It seemed they got only what was left over after all other health needs were addressed. And when we began establishing community group homes for mentally ill people, we ran into every roadblock imaginable—from neighborhood organizations and city council members to zoning laws hurriedly passed.

I have a vivid memory of stepping off the airplane in Valdosta, Georgia, on the way to a meeting about a planned group home, and being informed that the city council had voted the night before to deny approval. It was not a pleasant day!

It is significant to note, though, that although group homes for people with mental illness are nearly always opposed, once they are established and the community members get to know their "new neighbors," the stigma, almost without exception, vanishes. This happened in Valdosta, after we were eventually able to get permission to develop the home. The community soon just "adopted" the recovering patients, and the home became a model for other cities.

I hear about the problem of stigma over and over in the thousands of letters I have received from people who know about my interest in mental health. A young college student who wrote to me in the late 1970s summarized the dilemma quite well:

> Because I am aware that many people are truly ignorant when it comes to the subject of mental health, I have concealed that I am going to a therapist from most people. I do this not only to escape the fact that I might be labeled a "crazy" person but because I am twenty-one years old and will soon be looking for a job after I graduate from college next year. The fact that I have been emotionally ill might get in the way of finding a good job.
>
> I feel that if people were made aware of the widespread problem of mental illness and its true nature, and . . . that most people can be helped and even cured, then we all could start to be more open about mental illness and have people who need help receive it and be accepted by others as readily as they would be if they had a physical illness. After successful treatment they should be as able to lead normal and productive lives as they would if they had been cured of a physical disease.

I couldn't agree more. Yet, unfortunately, twenty-five years later, we as a society have still not reached that point. That is why I have decided to write this book. My goal for many years has been to see the stigma of mental illness eradicated. And I believe the more we educate ourselves, and the more we come to know our mentally ill neighbors, the closer we come to attaining that goal.

Today, science has made dramatic breakthroughs in our understanding of the causes and treatments of mental illnesses. We now know that many have hereditary and physical components, that they are not the result of a weak will or misguided parenting as we had once believed. If you or someone you love is suffering from mental illness, there is no reason to feel ashamed.

I am pleased to have this opportunity to write about these issues that have so absorbed me over the years and about the exciting developments in the field. I know there is still much to be learned and much that remains to be done if we are to continue to improve the quality of life for those who suffer, many in silence.

But today, there is help and hope for those with mental illness.

Chapter 1

A Mother's Lament . . .
And a Story of Hope

Recently I received a letter, as I so often do, from a woman whose family member is struggling with a mental illness. Alice wrote to thank me for my mental health work. She also mentioned that her local chapter of the National Alliance for the Mentally Ill (NAMI), an organization dedicated to supporting the interests of families and their mentally ill loved ones, was looking for volunteers who would be willing to inform the public about parents' concerns.

"I would love to be able to raise public awareness," Alice wrote, "but there's one big stumbling block. Each time I try to talk to groups about my daughter's fifteen-year struggle with schizophrenia, I cry.

"I cry most every night before I go to sleep," she continued. "I cry when I see street people. I cry when I think that even if a 'miracle' drug is produced, Stephanie will still have lost a part of her life. I cry when I think she's never gone to a dance with a boy; that she'll never marry; never be a mother; never experience life in the way others do.

"I cry when my older daughter gets to travel the world as a representative of her law firm while Stephanie sits on her bed and rocks. I cry when my middle daughter publishes articles in our local newspaper and Stephanie smokes and listens to her 'voices.'

"I cry for people in Somalia, in Bosnia, and now in Oklahoma City. But those who've lost loved ones there will grieve for months and years and eventually find peace. Those of us who have lost children to mental illness (and Stephanie is lost, even though she is alive) experience what one father aptly described as 'a funeral that never ends.' . . .

"I'd give anything if I could speak, or had some talent, some magic. But since that can't be, I and thousands like me will be ever grateful to you."

I feel privileged to be a voice for Alice and other individuals and families who have been affected by mental illness. I have witnessed firsthand their suffering and I have the deepest empathy for the anguish they have to endure every day of their lives.

As I pore through my mail and travel and talk to those who know of my interest in mental health, I constantly hear stories—stories of the emotionally disturbed child for whom no treatment program is available within the community; of the mother whose young adult son has been stricken with schizophrenia and spends his life in and out of the hospital and community programs; of the widow whose farmer-husband slowly withdrew from life into deep depression on the failing family farm; of the parents who have depleted their life savings and all of their resources in an effort to help their daughter who has manic-depression. I have seen the real suffering that cannot be captured by statistics or reflected in government reports.

But I am also aware that, although science has not yet discovered everything there is to know about mental illness, today there is so much we know and so much we can do. Almost everyone with a mental illness can be helped to lead a more normal life. We have learned that mental illnesses are not lifestyle choices, but rather that most of the major illnesses are diseases of the brain for which solutions are being sought and found.

To Alice and the millions of you who find yourselves in similar situations, and to the rest of us who may have a hard time comprehending the true nature of mental illness and its consequences, I offer this as a book of hope.

How I Became Involved

People aware of my long-standing commitment to mental health often ask if my involvement is based on personal experience, if my family had somehow been afflicted by the diseases on which I have worked for so many years. The answer is no, although during my childhood I did know a young man in Plains (Jimmy's cousin) who was in and out of the state mental institution, Central State Hospital in Milledgeville, Georgia. At that time I was still too unsophisticated to know whether he was suffering from manic-depression or schizophrenia or just what his problem was. His father had died and his mother tried to take care of him, but this was a long time ago, and I'm sure his mother lacked the resources or the knowledge to know what to do.

When Tommy was at home, I was afraid of him. When I heard him coming down the street, I would run and hide. Looking back, I don't know why I felt I had to get away, because he was never violent, just very nervous and loud.

Every so often, he would get really vocal, and everyone would know he was in trouble again. Soon the police would pick him up on the street, unceremoniously lay him across the backseat of their car, give him a shot, sometimes even handcuff him or put him in a straitjacket, and take him back to the hospital.

Tommy's condition and the way he was treated made a deep impression on me as a child. Later, after we were married, Jimmy and I visited him at the state hospital on several occasions.

But my true involvement with mental health did not begin until 1970, when I was working in Jimmy's campaign for governor of Georgia. My interest was piqued, I recall, by the many people who asked me: If your husband is elected, what will he do for my emotionally disturbed child? my depressed brother? my psychotic aunt?

And his own cousin?

Jimmy and I were on different schedules then, trying to reach as many people as possible. One day, I was surprised to learn that he was going to be in the same town I was later in the evening. So I stayed and went to his rally. He did not know I was there. When he was through speaking, I got in line with everybody else to shake hands with him.

As often happens in receiving lines, he reached out to take my hand while still talking with the person in front of me. Then he saw who I was, grinned, and asked, "What are you doing here?"

"I came to see what you are going to do about mental health when you are governor," I replied.

He smiled. "We're going to have the best system in the country," he said, "and I'm going to put you in charge of it."

He did not put me in charge of it, of course, but I did become a member, along with mental health professionals, laypeople, parents, and other concerned citizens, of the governor's commission he formed to improve services to the mentally and emotionally disabled.

Thus began my education about mental illness, and I had a lot to learn.

I went to all the meetings of the commission, volunteered once a week at the new Georgia Regional Hospital, and visited other regional hospitals, reporting back to the commission members—and to my husband—what I found. And I spoke out about the issue, trying to make it an acceptable subject of conversation.

My experience at Georgia Regional Hospital was especially revealing. I helped mentally disturbed children, planted flowers with geriatric patients, and followed up with alcoholics who had been put in the hospital to dry out. I fed some who needed help, read stories to others, and watched them all respond to attention.

But it was a struggle for me. One day, after I'd spent some time in a children's ward—trying to hold back tears all the while—the superintendent took me to his office and said, "I've watched you this morning, and I have to say one thing. If you're going to help at all, you've got to get over your tears. Don't let it get the best of you. We need you."

He was right, of course. But it was hard for me not to feel sorry for every child I saw, and for every adult, many of whom had been in institutions most of their lives. It was frustrating not to be able to unlock whatever it was inside that kept them from functioning properly and leading normal lives. After all, this was long before today's medications had been researched and developed.

Over time, I did acquire a sense of acceptance. And one thing I learned for sure was how dependent these people were on others, including me, to care for them. They couldn't care for themselves, and their families weren't always influential enough or in those days willing to speak out about mentally ill family members. The more I traveled on behalf of the commission and the longer I worked, the more I realized how much needed to be changed and how important this work could be.

Over the next four years, we made much progress in the mental health program in our state, moving patients from Central State Hospital into new, smaller regional hospitals and a few group homes, where we were able to get communities to accept them. This process of deinstitutionalization—the move from large institutions to community-based care—had been called for in the Community Mental Health Centers Act of 1963, and we hoped it would be a more humane way of caring for people with mental illnesses. In many instances, it was.

One day I visited patients who were being moved into a former air force base in Thomasville, Georgia, that had been converted into a regional hospital. On their very first day at the center, they would receive a welcoming letter from the mayor of the town. For many, this was the first mail they had ever received. And instead of having clothes passed out to them, as had been done in the larger institution, they were allowed to pick their own from little stores labeled "His" and "Hers." They could also choose their own food in a cafeteria line.

The staff in Thomasville had to teach the patients how to do these simple things, and even how to eat. At the larger institution, it had been easier just to feed them rather than take the time to help them feed themselves and then clean up after them. In so many ways, these newly released patients had to learn how to live again. They were like little children.

I remember watching two patients sitting on a step. They had just arrived from Central State Hospital and didn't know how to communicate. One wanted a puff from a cigarette the other held. He kept inching closer and closer until he finally touched his neighbor; without speaking, he motioned for what he wanted. But it would not be very many weeks before I saw the two of them wandering around together, talking with each other. They had been shut up and dominated for so long, it was amazing to see how they flourished when given a little freedom.

One weekend I drove to Ocilla, in a rural area of Georgia, to visit a community mental health center. There I saw the real human results of our efforts. An elderly man, who stuttered so badly that it was painful to listen to him, stands out in my mind. He told me, "I-I-I was the t-t-town crazy unt-t-il th-th-they opened th-th-this place." He had spent his life on the streets, taking handouts and causing trouble. But he had not missed a day at the center since it opened. He kept the yards swept and raked and helped inside the building. The staff told me they could not have gotten along without him.

When he was called on to sing during the afternoon program for visitors, he opened his mouth and the words of "How Great Thou Art" poured forth, clear and beautiful, without a single stutter. I cried.

Later, when we were in the White House, Jimmy established the President's Commission on Mental Health, and I was the honorary chairperson (anti-nepotism laws prevented my being chairperson). We were given one year to assess the current system and make recommendations from which new legislation could be drafted.

We needed the expert advice of professionals, but we also wanted the knowledge and wisdom of people from other fields and backgrounds because of our conviction that mental health problems are the problems of all citizens—ourselves, our families, our neighbors, and our friends. So perhaps our most important undertaking was our series of public hearings across the country. We listened for hours to hundreds of consumers, relatives of mentally ill people, advocates, psychiatrists, psychologists, social workers, laypersons, community leaders, and state and county officials as they related their firsthand experiences with the current system of care.

I still have vivid recollections of those hearings.

I remember one mother with a disabled child who lived in a state without facilities to care for her son's physical and emotional disabilities in, as she put it, "one ballgame"—one agency.

With proper care, she said, dealing with him as a whole child, he could have been rehabilitated within a couple of years. Without it, he would be institutionalized for the rest of his life, at a cost of hundreds of thousands of dollars to the state.

"What about the cost to society?" she asked me tearfully. "This is America that's being thrown down the drain if somebody doesn't help the emotionally disturbed child."

It was shocking to hear about the wasted lives of children. And equally shocking to hear about the failure of the mental health system to adequately serve other citizens because of where they lived, or who they were—their age, gender, race, or cultural background. Others were held back by their particular disability or economic circumstances.

And despite its humane goals, we learned that deinstitutionalization had a major failing: People were being turned out of institutions throughout the country without adequate community programs in place to support them. Over and over again we heard of the plight of individuals with severe and persistent mental illnesses who had been returned to their communities to lead marginal existences on the fringes of society—in and out of institutions, jobless, homeless, feared by almost everyone, and often hungry and despairing. Their problems pointed up critical weaknesses in our system: the lack of adequate planning and coordination of services between federal, state, and local programs; the blurred lines of responsibility and accountability; the treatment programs dictated by reimbursement mechanisms rather than by patients' needs.

Insurance was a problem then as now. Existing health insurance programs did not cover mental illnesses. Without adequate coverage, there was no incentive for people to overcome their fear of the stigma of mental illness and seek necessary psychiatric help.

We learned that populations with special needs were neglected. For example, although we know that the incidence of mental illness and emotional distress is higher among elderly citizens than the general population (see chapter 3), we found almost no outreach or in-home programs to bring senior citizens in contact with the services they needed. As a nation, we mostly relied on nursing homes, a dubious resource for good mental health care. Members of minority ethnic groups often felt intimidated or misunderstood by white mental health personnel. Fewer than 2 percent of the psychiatrists in our country were black, fewer still Hispanic, and only thirteen were Native Americans.

One day I visited the National Institute of Mental Health and learned that federal grants for research programs were wholly inadequate. I was told that just as the scientists were on the threshold of new discoveries about the brain, they were frustrated by cuts in funding for their research projects.

Programs directed at preventing mental illnesses were equally underfunded and marginalized. Why did the government always simply react to problems rather than help to avert them in the first place? As that mother who spoke out at the regional hearing so poignantly described, we allowed children to become really sick and in need of long-term care rather than take preventive action. In addition, too many children suffered from abuse and indifference, while others had severe learning disabilities. These problems, if neglected, could have profound mental health consequences.

Our commission prepared a set of recommendations based on the needs we had found, and we presented them to the President in an Oval Office ceremony in April 1978 (we *had* done it in one year!). We hoped that within the next ten years, our recommendations would bring about high-quality mental health care at reasonable cost to all who needed it.

We recommended changes in housing programs and in Medicare and Medicaid laws to provide adequate services for those with severe and persistent mental illness; "performance contracts" to make it easier for states to develop community mental health centers so that mentally ill people would not end up on the streets; health insurance coverage for mental illnesses; grants and loans to psychiatric students who would repay them by working in underserved areas; incentives for training in the special needs of minorities and ethnic groups, children and adolescents, the elderly, and women. We gave special emphasis to research and urged the establishment of an Office of Prevention within NIMH. We also recommended legislation aimed at protecting those who are mentally ill from a broad range of discriminatory practices, through an advocacy system and a special bill of rights.

And in May 1979, Jimmy submitted the Mental Health Systems Act to Congress. It passed and was funded a little more than a year later, in September 1980. We were jubilant!

Sadly, our elation was short-lived. Within a few weeks, Ronald Reagan was elected president, and with the change in administrations, many of our dreams were gone. Reagan's attitude toward the government's role in human services and mental health was not the same as ours, and having just been elected, he pushed his agenda through an overly passive Congress. Thus, the many facets of the Mental Health Systems Act were effectively nullified by the Omnibus Budget Reconciliation Act of 1981.

It was a bitter loss, but I have always been pleased about the commission and its recommendations, for they have served as a guide for many states that have adopted more humane, up-to-date policies. And some of its most significant principles were incorporated into new or existing federal programs throughout the 1980s.

Since we left the White House, I have been able to continue my work through a program at The Carter Center in Atlanta.

Our activities focus on stigma, children, and equity in mental health care. Also, beginning in 1985, we have had an annual symposium, bringing together national leaders in the mental health community to focus on a topic of common concern. We also have a task force of prominent individuals with whom we meet regularly and who provide direction for our activities.

The Changes I Have Witnessed

During the time I have been involved in mental health issues, so much has changed. Tremendous progress has been made in understanding the brain and the nature of mental illnesses, new medications have been developed, and treatment methods have improved dramatically. Mental illnesses are now definable, they can be diagnosed, and treatments are effective.

We have learned that for many people, mental illness is actually biologically based. There is now strong scientific evidence that some major illnesses such as schizophrenia, manic-depression (also called bipolar disorder), and obsessive-compulsive disorder are related to a genetic predisposition that causes people to develop the illness, and that structural or chemical problems in the brain are involved. For depression, a chemical imbalance in the body can be to blame in much the same way that abnormal levels of insulin occur with diabetes. With proper treatment, the imbalance can be corrected. Sometimes, several factors combine to bring on the illness. Environmental factors, for instance, and stressful life experiences can interact with our biological makeup to precipitate the illness.

The family and consumer movement is another major change. When Jimmy was governor in the early 1970s, there were only a few advocates in our state struggling to get better care for those who were suffering. No one wanted to be identified with the issue because of the stigma attached. It has only been in the last decade or so that families and consumers have "come out of the closet" and formed an influential lobby for better mental health services.

Over the last few years these changes have been reflected in the halls of Congress. Mental health became an integral part of the national debate over health care reform and received more visibility at a national level in 1994 than I have ever seen. In 1996 there was even legislation passed improving insurance coverage for mental illnesses. The legislation removed the traditionally lower caps on annual and lifetime coverage for these illnesses, requiring that they be the same as those for physical illnesses, but the legislation did not go far enough in providing equitable coverage. It was a small step, but a step in the right direction. We in the mental health community feel that *anything* that puts mental illness on a par with physical illness is a breakthrough.

The Tragedy of Stigma Has Not Changed

President John F. Kennedy once said, "The great enemy of truth is very often not the lies, deliberate, contrived, and dishonest, but the myths, persistent, persuasive, and unrealistic." This is especially true when we consider mental illness.

The overwhelming majority of people with mental illnesses are capable of leading normal lives—of living at home, going to school, working, being productive, tax-paying citizens. Even among those who are homeless, according to a federal task force report, only 5 to 7 percent need to be in special living situations. There is no reason for anyone to be ashamed of having a mental illness, and yet many feel that way and suffer unwarranted discrimination due to the associated stigma. The dictionary describes stigma as "a mark of disgrace or reproach," but for those who experience it, it is indescribable—and devastating.

Our society has great difficulty in talking about and dealing with mental illnesses. While there has been some improvement in the past decade as we have learned more about causes and treatments, the stigma—based on myth and misinformation—is still enormous and pervasive. For example, it is a myth that mental illness makes people violent and evil monsters. It is true that a very small percentage of those with the serious illnesses who do not receive proper treatment are dangerous, especially when also using alcohol or drugs. But the stereotype of the mentally ill person as violent is erroneous. As the American Psychiatric Association explains, "People with mental illnesses—like other people with disabilities—are far more likely to be victims of crime than they are to be criminals." Those who are afflicted tend to be more passive and withdrawn and are especially vulnerable.

Kathy Cronkite, daughter of television journalist Walter Cronkite and an accomplished talk show host, journalist, and writer, has suffered from severe depression. At a Conversations at The Carter Center program on "Coping with the Stigma of Mental Illness" in April 1996, she spoke of her own struggles with the myths and stigma. "I felt so ashamed," she explained to the audience of about four hundred Atlantans. "I kept my illness and medications a secret. Part of the stigma came from within— from my own sense of failure. I was afraid that if my friends found out, they would pussyfoot around me. I was afraid of losing credibility and my job. I was afraid people would think I was weak or crazy."

Kathy Cronkite's fears are not so far-fetched. In 1992, the Alliance for the Mentally Ill of Pennsylvania conducted a statewide telephone survey to assess how that state's residents view persons with mental illness. Forty percent of the 350 respondents believed that "most people who are mentally ill could be well if they only had the will," and 93 percent agreed that people who have different types of mental illness are discriminated against by others. Those who had observed such discrimination in their communities reported witnessing verbal abuse and ridicule directed toward mentally ill individuals or discriminatory hiring practices once the condition became known to an employer.

This is tragic, and it affects the lives of so many. Statistics from the National Institute of Mental Health indicate just how widespread mental illness is.* In any given year, more than 50 million people, or 22 percent of our nation's population over age eighteen, will suffer a mental disorder, and an estimated 12 percent or 7.5 million children will be affected. That's almost a third more than the 20 percent of Americans who suffer from cardiovascular disease. And scientists report that 90 percent of those with mental illness can be helped using new therapies. Yet only about 30 percent ever receive treatment. Stigma plays a major role in keeping those who are afflicted from obtaining the help they desperately need.

The indirect costs of mental illness (costs unrelated to psychiatric or medical care, such as social disruptions, unemployment, and loss of productivity), estimated at $75 billion in 1990, are the same as those associated with heart disease. In the United States, depression alone accounts for more people out of work and in bed than any other disorder except cardiovascular disease.

---

* The numerous statistics cited in this book are drawn from various sources. Some may appear inconsistent because of the way different surveys and research studies are conducted. For example, one study might include people between the ages of eighteen and fifty-five, while another might investigate individuals between the ages of fifteen and seventy.

But there is a huge difference in perception—heart disease is "acceptable," mental illness is not. Although some experts put the indirect and direct costs of mental illness as high as $150 billion annually, the human costs—the poverty, the broken homes and lives, the isolation, the loss of self-esteem, the suffering caused by negative stereotypes—cannot be measured.

I've been distressed to hear from so many people with mental illness who have found themselves virtually shunned when they disclosed their problem to others. People don't know how to talk to them or often will deliberately avoid them. As one person said, "They see you coming and turn and go a different way." How can one measure the degree to which such stigma adds insult to injury?

In a larger context, these stereotypes and the accompanying stigma affect the way our nation as a whole deals with and treats its mentally ill population.

The Scope of the Problem

In part, because of the stigma associated with it, the true impact of mental illness on our society and even the world is often nearly invisible. A landmark 1990 assessment of the global burden of disease by the Harvard School of Public Health, the World Health Organization, and the World Bank found that of the ten leading causes of disability (when measured in years lived with the disability) in the world, half were psychiatric conditions—depression, alcohol use, manic depression, schizophrenia, and obsessive-compulsive disorder. It also determined that by the year 2020, the leading cause of disability in the world will be major depression.

According to Christopher J. L. Murray, associate professor of international health economics at Harvard University, and

Alan D. Lopez of the World Health Organization in Geneva, Switzerland, who edited the study, "The burdens of mental illnesses have been seriously underestimated by traditional approaches that take account only of deaths and not disability. While psychiatric conditions are responsible for little more than 1 percent of deaths, they account for almost 11 percent of disease burden worldwide."

In a visit to The Carter Center in May 1993, Dr. Murray talked about the report at a meeting of our mental health task force. He told us that he and the scientists who worked with him were amazed at the findings of the study. "As a nonpsychiatrist," he said, "I had always been skeptical of the claims I heard from the psychiatric community about how psychiatric disorders were neglected, so from that starting point, the results were even more surprising."

I don't want to overwhelm you with statistics, but I think a few other key findings will help you understand the scope of the problem we are facing. The alarming facts about mental health care and the attitudes associated with mental illness in our country today attest to the burden in human as well as financial terms.

• Eighty percent of those with persistent, severe mental disorders are unemployed today, although with proper treatment and rehabilitation many of them are capable of working.[1]

• The National Alliance for the Mentally Ill (NAMI) has found that more than 7.5 percent of people held in the nation's jails suffer from severe mental disorders.

• Research has shown that depression in the elderly has grave medical consequences, nearly tripling the rate of strokes and significantly increasing the risk for heart attacks, hip fractures, and severe infections. Yet, according to the National Institute of Mental Health, while nearly 8 percent of older Americans have symptoms of depression severe enough to warrant treatment, about 63 percent of this group receive none. For those residing in nursing homes, the rate of mental disorder is much higher—nearly two thirds have symptoms that require treatment, yet 90 percent of them do not receive it.

• A 1992 study by the Federal Task Force on Homelessness and Mental Illness found that approximately one third of the single adult homeless population suffer from a severe mental illness, frequently co-occurring with alcohol and drug abuse.

• Unrecognized mental disorders account for 30 to 80 percent of all cases that primary care physicians see in their offices, according to Dr. Kelly Kelleher of the Mental Health Policy Resource Center in Washington, D.C. These physicians often have too little time or training to be able to diagnose or effectively treat mental illnesses. Besides the human suffering this creates, lack of access to mental health professionals can also waste valuable resources. For example, unnecessary angiograms for individuals suffering from panic disorders (who think their chest pains and breathing difficulties are really heart attacks) cost an estimated $33 million a year.

• Suicide is the ninth leading cause of death in the United States, according to the National Institute of Mental Health. Research has shown that nearly all of those who commit suicide have a diagnosable mental illness or substance abuse disorder, or both. With treatment, the tragedy of suicide is often preventable.

• While recent legislation has brought about some change, mental illnesses are still not covered by insurance on a parity with physical illnesses. I have worked hard to correct this for many years, because it is so unfair. Even my family's insurance plan with Emory University, which, comparatively speaking, is a very good one, limits inpatient treatment for mental health to only sixty days a year, while there is no limit on the number of days of hospitalization for a physical ailment. In addition, the number of visits to a counselor are sharply limited when compared to unrestricted visits to other health care professionals. And the co-payments for mental illnesses are much higher than those for physical illnesses.

One irate consumer wrote in a letter to *USA Today*, "If insurance companies don't consider mental illness an illness, how do you expect the public to perceive it?" I agree with her wholeheartedly. I firmly believe that making insurance benefits for mental illnesses and physical illnesses the same would do more than anything to dispel stigma.

As we have seen from the above facts and statistics, undiagnosed and untreated mental illnesses create staggering costs in our society. Yet, in another indication of our attitudes, the expenditures for mental health care in our country have traditionally averaged only about 10 to 12 percent of total health care costs. Those who suffer from these illnesses encounter discrimination in so many ways.

A. M. Rosenthal described the problem quite succinctly when he wrote in *The New York Times* in January 1995, "If a person breaks a leg in the street, civil help tends to him quickly—ambulance, doctors, police. Break your mind and you lie there. The American community finds money for taking care of tens of millions—the poor, the aged, the physically ill. Why are there so many mentally ill people cut off from help?" Stigma is at the root of this and so many other problems relating to the care of persons suffering from mental illnesses. But I believe this all can change.

How do we fight stigma? Through education. It has been my experience that when people understand mental illnesses, the stigma vanishes. Therefore, I want to share what I have learned about the nature of these disorders and the great strides now being made in treatment. Shedding light on misperceptions that are based on "myth—persistent, persuasive, and unrealistic" is the best way I know to end them.

A Story of Hope

Sometimes it's hard to grasp the impact of a long list of statistics. What does all of this really mean to you, to your friends and neighbors, to your family? The numbers make more sense when we put a human face to them. And that's why I've decided to share Angela Koppenol's story with you.

Angela, like 17 million other Americans, suffers from major depression. I first learned of her battle with this disease and with borderline personality disorder when a profile of her life appeared in the *Macon* (Ga.) *Telegraph* in October 1996. Angela had been interviewed for an article publicizing the free depression screenings available across the country during National Mental Illness Awareness Week, which is usually the first full week in October. What drew my interest was this young woman's dedication to helping others in the same situation. "If I can do anything by being honest about my own problems," she had said, "I hope I can help everyone understand that those who suffer from mental illnesses are ordinary people with a disease. . . . It's no different from cancer—it's something that just happens."

In a lengthy phone call with me later that month, Angela shared with great sincerity and clarity much about her illness and recovery. Angela speaks for millions of other individuals caught in the same situation—and she speaks with anguish and with hope.

"I feel sensitive about mental illness," she said, "because I went undiagnosed and untreated for quite a while. I guess in the back of my mind, I knew I had an illness. I knew I was just so different from so many people around me. They all seemed so happy, and I knew that I never was.

"Actually, I blamed God a lot, even though I went to worship and was very involved with my church. I felt that somehow I was so bad somewhere in my life that God must have been punishing me with being so unhappy all the time and suicidal.

"I found ways to hide my illness, I guess because I was afraid. You hear the news stories that people who have mental illness are always violent. You hear the jokes that they're always stupid, and they're going to go off at any minute and harm you. Although I never felt harmful toward anyone else, I knew I felt harmful toward me. I was very afraid of what people would say or think about me.

"In fact, that extended to my whole family. I had an aunt who was mentally ill for years, although I think she's better now. Even growing up, my mother always made sure that we understood that this particular aunt was not really sick. She was just doing everything she did, including a suicide attempt, for attention.

"So I got the idea real early that people who have mental illness actually are faking it, usually for attention. I was afraid to get treatment because I was afraid my family would feel that I was faking it too. I found ways to hide a lot of my symptoms."

Angela's borderline personality disorder caused her to have narrow views of people and that created great difficulties in making friends. "I knew when I was very, very young that I did not have many friends . . . and the friends I did have, I was finding ways to sabotage the relationships. People were either extremely good and almost godlike or something they did to me was so terrible, I just could not associate with them. That caused a real strain on relationships."

As a result, she would often isolate herself. "I can remember as a youth, my father coming into my room saying, 'Why don't you come join the family? Why don't you watch TV with us?' I'd always have a library book propped open on the bed. I spent a huge amount of time reading. Your book friends are your real friends, I felt, because they wouldn't do anything to you. You were just reading about them. I always did have some excuse for why I really just couldn't spend a lot of time with the family.

"The times that I did spend with them, even those relationships were extremely unstable. My ideas of who I was were extremely unstable. I could not see myself as a good person, although I tried harder than anything to be a perfect person— to do everything perfectly, and to make myself somehow worthy of leading a happy life. A real compulsive effort to be perfect was a large part of my problem early on."

Ironically, that desire for perfection made Angela an excellent employee. "I went into bookkeeping, which is a field you have to be perfect in," she explained. "The numbers have to match up in just the right spot at the end of the day. They can't be off. You have to have your filing just so, so you can lay your hands on invoices. Even in working with computers, the paper has to be perfectly lined up so you get the whole report on it.

"The field I chose actually aided that need, that horrible need to be perfect. Somehow if I could just be perfect enough, the terrible things I felt would disappear, or I would be rewarded in some way for them. Maybe even if it was just a little praise from my bosses, that would be enough. Often, that went further than the raises I got. The raises helped financially, but mostly what helped was getting a little something that would tell me that surely I wasn't as bad as I thought I was."

Although her bookkeeping job helped Angela a great deal, at the same time, it continued to put extra stress on her. "If occasionally something went wrong, or if I needed correction, I was afraid that it would reaffirm I was a bad and horrible person. Criticism was extremely excruciating. And often, even if it wasn't criticism of me, if it was just a change in policy, I would think it was a change because of something I had done. I would feel suicidal after that, and that was a struggle."

In 1986, when she was about twenty-three, Angela first attempted suicide. "I took pills," she admitted openly. "It's not as easy to kill the body as it is to kill the soul. I thought a big handful was more than enough, but I survived through the night. I had just been attacked a month or so before by a rapist. I got away, and it turned out to be just a purse snatching. But later, I was interviewed by the police, and my description matched the description of several other women in our small community who had recently been raped."

That trauma and the pressure of having to move back in with her parents made Angela feel as if everything had failed her. "I wasn't living on my own anymore, and I was devastated by it all.

"When you're mentally ill," Angela explained, "you're living in the darkest, most horrible place, and you're living there alone. Mental illness makes you feel devoid of meaning; it makes you feel devoid of hope. And the loss of hope is one of the most tremendous losses for people who suffer mental illness. The whole view of yourself and the world around you becomes so dark, and so hard. It's an incredible place to find yourself. You just want relief. Your whole focus becomes how can I get someone to make me well? What can I do to not feel like this anymore?"

Angela's first suicide attempt was a cry for help. It had taken her ten years to begin to ask for the relief she needed, and it would be many more still before she actually found it.

"I developed a lot of symptoms such as self-mutilation. It was a way of releasing myself from the pain and punishing myself for not being able to do what other people do and live the kind of life I thought I could lead. I thought I really don't want to live with the pain of the mental illness. So maybe if I cause myself some physical pain, God will let me do that instead."

After many more suicide attempts and hospitalizations, Angela found the right treatment in 1993. "The psychiatrist who was treating me was a very compassionate man. He was willing to listen to me and didn't force me to stay on medications that didn't work. We finally tried an older medication, Desyrel.

"With the Desyrel, I started noticing some stability. Thank God Almighty, for me it did not have a lot of side effects. Most of mine went away with treatment. We played with the dose a little bit until we found a comfortable one. I've been on it for two to three years."

The medication keeps Angela stable now on a day-to-day basis, but when she's under severe stress, her symptoms will flare up again. "So, I have learned how to watch my stress and my symptom levels and when I need to back off my schedule, I can do that and prevent getting sicker. I say to myself, 'You're getting into a red zone here and you don't want to be there anymore.' So I can back away. That has given me the feeling of having some control. I know I'll never have total control because this is an illness that I developed very early and the likelihood that it will go away totally and that I'll never need treatment again is unrealistic."

Despite her continuing struggles, Angela feels that she has recovered to a great extent.

"For the most part, I live a very normal life now," she said. "I don't consider myself well. I consider myself . . . what do cancer patients call it? I'm in remission. But I'm doing better than I ever have. In fact, I am no longer plagued with depression. I'm basically happy. I've held the same part-time job for four years. I'm married. I never thought I could sustain a relationship like a marriage, but I have been married for five years now to a loving, understanding husband. I never expected to live to the age of thirty. I was fully convinced that I would be dead long before then. You can't imagine my surprise and delight when I actually turned thirty years old. And this year, I turned thirty-three. I'm a three-year survivor beyond what I thought I'd ever be.

"I actually have plans for a year from now and for five years and goals that I want to meet. I have more hope in a single day now than I have ever had in all my years put together.

"It's a remarkable change. At least now I feel that usually I walk in the light. I only have to walk in the shadows for a short time."

May Angela's struggle be a source of inspiration and hope to us all.

Chapter 2

What Is Mental Illness?

Mental illness seems such a broad topic, one that is difficult to get our arms around. And until just a few years ago, it was also a subject shrouded in mystery and fear. As recently as the 1960s, researchers and clinicians still had not developed ways to distinguish one mental illness from another. If these conditions were difficult to diagnose, imagine how difficult it was to treat them. Even when I began working in the field, in the early 1970s, the general practice was to shuttle an afflicted one off to an institution. Fortunately, things have changed. These disorders can now be diagnosed and treated as accurately as other medical conditions.

Mental illnesses are illnesses that affect the way a person thinks, acts, and feels. Like most illnesses, they have intertwined biological, psychological, and environmental roots.[1] The more severe mental illnesses are primarily diseases of the brain that cause distorted thinking, feelings, or behavior. Just as there are many physical illnesses, there are a range of these disorders. They include the following:

• *Schizophrenia.* A major disorder in which there are disturbances in thoughts and emotions accompanied by delusions and hallucinations, distortions of language and communication, content of thought, perception, affect (emotion), sense of self, relationship to the external world, self-control and/or motor behavior. Schizophrenia is particularly disabling, generally interfering with the ability to work, relate to others, and take care of oneself.

• *Mood Disorders.* Clinical or major depression, mania (elation), and manic-depressive (bipolar) illness are referred to as mood disorders. Unlike the normal "down" mood that everyone experiences at times, *major depression* lingers on, and the sadness, dejection, and despair become more pronounced than warranted by the events of daily living. *Mania,* by contrast, is marked by an elation, abnormal excitability, exaggerated feelings of well-being, flight of ideas, excessive activity. Those suffering from *manic-depression* alternate between episodes of mania and major depression.

• *Anxiety Disorders.* A group of illnesses in which anxiety is the most prominent feature or in which anxiety appears when the affected persons try to resist symptoms such as phobias (abnormal fears), obsessions (persistent thoughts), or compulsions (irresistible impulses to do something). This is anxiety out of proportion to any identifiable reason or cause, a state of almost constant tension and fear. The two most common illnesses of this group are panic disorder, in which affected people are subject to attacks of panic from no discernible cause, and obsessive-compulsive disorder (OCD), in which affected persons have repetitive thoughts and behaviors that are difficult if not impossible to control.

The term *psychosis* is often used when describing severe mental illnesses. It refers to a mental state in which an individual's perception of reality is impaired. He or she may hallucinate (seeing, hearing, or even smelling things that aren't there), become incoherent and delusional (believing in something false or unreal), and may display bizarre behavior. Psychosis is a symptom of schizophrenia but may also occur with major depression and bipolar illness.

Schizophrenia, major depression and manic-depression, and some of the anxiety disorders are the most prevalent and disabling mental illnesses in our society, and are the ones that I will be focusing on in this book.

Mental retardation, by the way, is quite distinct from and should not be confused with mental illness. The former refers to pervasive intellectual impairment—the inability to learn normally and become fully independent. Mental retardation is a developmental disorder that can result from autism (see appendix A), Down's syndrome, lack of stimulation, or other developmental insults. A person with a mental illness is not intellectually impaired, and indeed can be quite intelligent. Writers William Styron, Art Buchwald, Ernest Hemingway, and Sylvia Plath all experienced depression, yet are examples of talented, even brilliant minds.

All of us experience brief periods of confusion, anxiety, or sadness as a normal part of our everyday lives. This is not mental illness. To qualify as a mental illness, the symptoms must be intense enough to interfere with normal functioning: sleeping, eating, social relationships, work, and maintaining appropriate behavior. One in five people in our nation have or will have a mental illness sometime in their lives. About 3 percent—five million adults—are considered to have severe and persistent mental illness. Before we delve into the symptoms of each of these conditions, let's explore what is believed to cause the onset of an episode of mental illness.

What Triggers Mental Illness?

Angela Koppenol spoke to me about the impact of extraordinary stress on her illness. She now knows to recognize when she's nearing her "red zone" and how to deal with it. Her experience illustrates current thinking about the origins of mental illnesses.

It is helpful to think of the onset and course of these diseases as being dependent on two interrelated factors:

• One's inborn vulnerability to a particular condition
• Environmental stress

For example, Angela might well have had a genetic predisposition to depression, which is strongly suggested by the fact that her aunt also suffered from the illness. That would be her inborn vulnerability. She certainly had an inclination for negative, pessimistic thoughts. The stress associated with the trauma of the assault and her return to her parents' home—which, at the age of twenty-three, was very difficult for her—may have pushed her into a full-blown depressive episode.

These two factors, vulnerability and stress, complement each other. When both are present, they can trigger the disorder. Had Angela not had the genetic predisposition for depression, the mugging might have been a terrible event in her life, but in time the memory might have faded without spurring a self-destructive reaction. By the same token, had Angela been spared the assault, perhaps she might never have made that first suicide attempt.

Scientists have found that a person who has a strong physiological vulnerability to mental illness requires relatively little environmental stress to provoke an episode. Think of Angela's intense reaction to on-the-job criticism. When the stress subsided, so did the symptoms; remember how she felt comforted when praised. Yet the symptoms may return with the next upsetting event.

For some individuals with severe disorders, it seems to take less and less stress, in a sort of kindling effect, to trigger each successive episode. The brain becomes accustomed to responding to tension in a certain way and does so with increasing ease, unless therapy and/or medication intervene.

For reasons still not fully understood, mental illnesses often begin to appear during late adolescence and early adulthood. Perhaps the maturing of the brain tips the scales, or the normal stresses and strains of this developmental stage combined with an individual's inborn vulnerability. Whatever the cause, their appearance—sometimes sudden, sometimes gradual—leaves family members, friends, and the victims themselves baffled and distraught.

Schizophrenia

Don Richardson found himself in just such a position. A former assistant superintendent of schools for the sprawling Los Angeles Unified School District and one of the co-founders of the National Alliance for the Mentally Ill, Don is also an adviser to our Carter Center mental health program.

"Our older son was a model student," he explained to me one day. "Everything he did was right. He was an Eagle Scout; he was a good scholar. He would go to his room to study without having been told. As we look back on it, however, many of these signs were symbolic of his illness. He became more and more of a loner. He became more difficult to talk with. We thought this was all part of the growth process. Since he was our oldest, we didn't have the experience of prior children."

Don's son went to college at the University of California at Santa Barbara and at Berkeley. "During that four-year period," Don continued, "we had the occasional visits and they went very well. He continued to do excellent work in college. As far as we were concerned, he was getting along all right until we got that phone call. That was our introduction, and from there on . . ."

The call came in 1972. Don's son had just graduated from Berkeley and had moved to the Silicon Valley to work in the burgeoning computer industry. "One day we got a call from a hospital in San Jose. Our son was in the hospital; he had been picked up by the police because he was in a restaurant, trying to jab his eyes out with a fork. He was having visual hallucinations. That was our introduction to mental illness. He was away from home during the traditional time when mental illness begins to show up in various behaviors, so we were not able to see these symptoms. As a result, it was a total bombshell when it hit us."

The Richardsons were not allowed this naïveté with their third child. "Our youngest son, Bill, began to show signs that we now recognized as mental illness as early as junior high school. We were convinced that it was drug-related, and it was. We now call this dual diagnosis [a combination of mental illness and substance abuse], but at that time, he was an adolescent experimenting and dealing in heavy drugs. He managed to get through high school with a lot of parental encouragement. My wife and I took turns constantly supervising him, and then one day, after thirty hours of constant talking and hallucinating and running out the door, he grabbed an ax and began destroying his room. He heard voices in the walls and wanted to find where they came from. This resulted in his first hospitalization. As of today, he has been involuntarily hospitalized forty-two times over a period of twenty-five years. He's the one who is the acting-out person. The more psychotic our oldest became, the more withdrawn he was. With the youngest, the more psychotic, the more visible, the more outgoing, and the more aggressive. We did experience the total cycle of his illness because he was at home at the time this was happening."

The Richardsons decided they would use whatever knowledge they had gathered in helping their sons to comfort the millions of others who were also suffering because of family members with mental illness. Their experience encouraged them to retire as early as possible and to devote the rest of their lives to discovering what mental illness is and working to eliminate it. That's when they became involved in the creation of NAMI and in their many other pursuits related to mental illness.

Schizophrenia is the most complex and puzzling of all the mental illnesses, and the most debilitating. It affects about 1 percent of the population, and afflicts men and women equally. About one hundred thousand new cases are diagnosed in this country annually. Because of its early onset (in the late teens or early adulthood) and the possibility of lifelong disability, its effect on families like the Richardsons, and perhaps yours, is catastrophic.

Contrary to popular belief, schizophrenia does not mean "split personality" or "multiple personality." Rather, the illness is a brain disease that can affect nearly every aspect of an individual's functioning. Particularly disabling, it causes disordered sensory perceptions and thinking and, as we have seen with Don's sons, it can manifest itself in different ways. While some sufferers become quiet, anxious, and withdrawn, their emotions dulled, others become aggressive and outspoken.

People in an acute phase of schizophrenia are said to be psychotic—out of touch with reality or unable to separate real from unreal experiences. Some may have only one such psychotic episode in a lifetime; others have many but lead relatively normal lives during the interim periods. Unfortunately, for some, schizophrenia is a chronic disorder that affects them for life.

The Symptoms of Schizophrenia

Those suffering from schizophrenia may experience:

• *Disordered Thinking.* They may be unable to "think straight" for hours on end; their thoughts may come in rapid-fire succession without logical sequence; their sentences may be fragmentary or jumbled.

• *Hallucinations.* If they have auditory hallucinations, they may hear voices telling them what to do or what not to do, voices that warn of danger, insult the individual, dictate, or describe activities. If they have visual hallucinations, victims may also see things that the rest of us don't see, which for them are very real.

• *Delusions.* Affected persons may entertain false beliefs. They may think that the radio is broadcasting their thoughts or that extraterrestrial aliens are controlling their behavior. The beliefs may be of grandeur (seeing oneself as Jesus or Napoleon), or they may be of persecution and paranoia (viewing a simple box of chocolates offered in friendship as if it were poison).

• *Inappropriate Emotions.* People with schizophrenia may laugh when they should be crying or cry when they should be laughing, or at times, show no emotion at all.

• *Withdrawal.* They may experience emotional and social withdrawal, lack of motivation, reduced language and emotional expressiveness. These can seriously impair personal relationships.

These symptoms of schizophrenia are divided into two categories: positive and negative. The positive symptoms include the hallucinations, delusions, and disordered thinking; the negative include emotional and social withdrawal, lack of motivation, and a limited ability to communicate or express emotion—in other words, a decrease or absence of normal, spontaneous feelings and behaviors.

Depression

Rod Steiger is an Academy Award–winning actor who has had starring roles in more than seventy-two films including *On the Waterfront* (for which he was nominated for an Oscar), *In the Heat of the Night* (for which he received one), *Oklahoma!,* and *Doctor Zhivago.* He has also been clinically depressed. In April 1996, he joined Kathy Cronkite at Conversations at The Carter Center to share his deeply felt emotions about his own depression.

Rod spoke with such conviction, such passion that at times we in the audience held our breaths and could only listen in stunned silence as he helped us get inside the very experience of depression. I would like to share some of his remarks with you.

"I have a clinical depression," he began matter-of-factly, "which is a chemical imbalance of the brain. It's a disease, like diabetes. And if I don't take my medicine in the morning, and I don't take it at night, I'll be great for about two weeks and then all of a sudden it'll start. It's very insidious, the way it starts.

"Somebody says, 'Where's the phone?'

" 'Over there!' " He growled, imitating his brusque overreaction to an innocent question.

"And I say to myself, What the hell is wrong with me? What am I getting angry about?

" 'Are you up?'

" 'Do I look like I'm lying down?' And then it starts to go down from there," he said.

Rod paused for a moment at the lectern and unfolded some pages he had written. "I wrote this in the midst of this torturous existence for my wife as well as my son . . . I'd like to read it to you.

"I want to die," he began reading in a steady voice that slowly built in cadence. "I don't want to move. I have no feeling for movement. To be left alone. To disappear. Not to be bothered with washing, shaving, talking, walking, going to the bathroom. If only to get out of this tunnel and the heavy darkness, cold and oily, constantly pressing against my brain and being . . ."

He continued, explaining his torture. And then he turned to a passage about his acting and the paralyzing fear of not being able to remember his lines "with everybody watching . . . even the rat in the corner of the saloon in the studio set is watching!

"I won't be able to do it," he said quickly. "I will not be able to remember. They're going to discover I am inadequate. I am unable," he said, beginning to cry. "I am weak."

"I must not scream. I must not scream in front of them. I must stay. I must not, must not listen to what's left of my mind. I must not, I must not run off the set. I must not run. I must not run. . . . They're going to find out that I'm weak. They'll find out I'm in pain. Oh God.

"What God?" he thundered. He paused. Then in a small voice he whispered, "I'll break down. I'll look like a fool, an idiot, and they'll find out. I can't act," and he wept again.

"But wait," Rod whispered. "There is a way out. You get a gun, a nice cool gun and . . ."

And in graphic terms he described just how he would end his life "without leaving behind a mess . . . blood on the walls, the carpet, the flowers, all over the cat . . . I'll get a small rowboat . . . I'll lower myself over the side, hold onto the boat with one hand, put the cool gun in my mouth with the other, and pull the trigger. No mess—fish food."

It was chilling.

And it was clear that Rod was not acting. In the retelling of his years battling untreated depression, he began reliving the experience before our eyes, and what a powerful experience it was. After he finished there was a moment of silence as if we in the audience needed to let his words sink in, as if we needed to catch our breaths before erupting in applause. What a courageous man!

Depression such as Rod's, which is called clinical or major depression, affects 17 million Americans every year. One in four women and one in ten men will develop the illness at some time in their lives. It can strike at any age, and the pain and suffering it causes—for those who have the illness and for those who care about them—cannot be overestimated. It can destroy family life as well as the life of the ill person.

And perhaps the saddest fact about depression is that so many people suffer needlessly. Only one in three will seek treatment, although the great majority—even those with the most severe disorders—can be helped. This is especially tragic because, with the treatments that are available, 80 percent of the people with serious depression can improve and return to daily activities, usually in a matter of weeks. Another distressing fact is that, according to the American Psychiatric Association, depression lies at the root of most suicides in our country.

Depressive disorders come in different forms, just as do other illnesses, such as heart disease. Major depression, as described above, is one of the most prevalent, with disabling episodes that can occur once, twice, or several times in a lifetime. Another form, which I will discuss later in this chapter, is manic-depressive illness.

The Symptoms of Depression

Rod is right. He does suffer from a disease. Major depression is neither a sign of personal weakness nor a condition that one can simply "snap out of." It is a very real and common illness that affects more than just the mind. But first, it is important to distinguish between clinical or major depression and normal sadness or "the blues."

All of us have moments when we are down. The loss of a loved one, a setback at work, any major difficulty can make us feel sad and blue for a while. This is normal. In depression, however, these feelings of sadness and hopelessness just don't go away.

The illness not only alters and disrupts one's mood, it also affects one's thoughts, body, and behavior. An individual's entire being is affected. Let's look at some of the potential symptoms more closely.

• *Mood.* A depressed individual may feel melancholy, sad, and miserable most of the time, with the loss of pleasure and interest in life. This can result in decreased energy, fatigue, fits of weeping or constantly feeling like crying, and an unusually high degree of irritability.

Rod Steiger's illness certainly reflected these symptoms. His agitation, exhaustion, and despair seemed overwhelming.

• *Thoughts.* Stubbornly negative, hopeless thoughts about the present and future dominate during depression, along with anxiety and dread out of proportion to actual events. Research shows that more than 60 percent of depressed people feel intense anxiety similar to what Rod described with respect to his acting abilities. They may have difficulty concentrating and making decisions; experience feelings of guilt, self-loathing, or worthlessness; and be preoccupied with death and suicidal thoughts or attempts.

• *Body.* Depression is also a physical illness. Affected individuals may experience disruptions in their normal eating and sleep patterns. Some are unable to sleep at all, or awaken very early in the morning. Others may sleep many more hours than usual.

In his book *The Good News About Depression,* Dr. Mark S. Gold states: "Depressed people also get less overall deep sleep, which is the most restorative and refreshing of all." Perhaps this is why someone who is depressed may spend long hours sleeping but still wake feeling exhausted and spent.

A loss of appetite and an accompanying loss of weight without dieting are common symptoms, as is sudden overeating.

The depressed individual may lose interest in sex, suffer from headaches or stomachaches, and complain of vague, mysterious physical pain that seems to migrate to different parts of the body.

• *Behavior.* Lethargy, an inability to get work done, and difficulty in reading or studying are all symptoms of depression. In addition, it may take great effort for those who are depressed to accomplish simple tasks such as washing, dressing, and eating. They may act restless, agitated, or jittery; experience slowed thoughts, movements, and speech; walk with a stooped and shuffling gait; or suddenly become extremely dependent.

For some people the symptoms of depression seem to have no obvious cause, and they endure even in the face of joyful events. People with depression may lack the energy to reach out for help, or they may feel so despondent that they believe any attempt to relieve their suffering will be fruitless.

Not everyone who is depressed will experience all of these symptoms. Some people experience a few, some many. Also, the severity of symptoms will vary with the individual.

Manic-Depressive Illness

One of my neighbors in Plains, Braxton Mallard, a man of about sixty, suffers from manic-depressive illness. One morning, while getting medicine for my mother, I ran into him at the drugstore. The pharmacist in Plains has been helpful to Braxton, giving him literature to read about his illness and providing him with part-time work running errands.

Since I was researching this book, I invited Braxton to my office to talk to me about his illness. He was eager to share his story "if this will help somebody." And so he began an account of his condition. "I was aware that I had some problems," he said, settling into the couch, facing me. "But it wasn't until I was in my thirties that I realized I was different. A lot of people picked on me. I took a lot of things wrong. After I went in the service, I noticed I was a loner."

A highly decorated member of the peacetime military, Braxton realized that he was ill while stationed in Korea at a nuclear weapons depot. "I was going into a deep depression. I knew that there was something wrong. I took so much Valium. I went to doctors and it was prescribed. I'd go to one doctor, then go to another doctor. I was eating Valium to kill the pain. I had migraine headaches. I believed I had bursitis. In those years the bursitis kept increasing and I kept increasing the drugs.

"One day, I got fed up with the things I was seeing that were going on around me. I guess I was a perfectionist. I had a bottle of Valium and swallowed all of it. One of the NCOs [non-commissioned officers] found me."

Braxton was taken to a military hospital in Korea and diagnosed as having manic-depression with suicidal tendencies. "I don't run from this illness," he told me. "I know I've got it, and I know what I am."

Others, however, have run from their illness. Actress Margot Kidder made that clear in a recent television interview with Barbara Walters after a bizarre incident in Los Angeles and her diagnosis of manic-depressive illness made the headlines. "I hid by taking drugs," she told Walters during the interview at the actress's home in Montana. "I hid by getting drunk. I hid by literally hiding in my house and not going out and not picking up the phone. I hid by all manner of deceit in the same way that a gay man hides his gayness before he is able to come out of the closet. The hiding has taken such an extraordinary toll, as much as the illness itself."

Unlike depression, which can strike at any time, manic-depression usually begins during adolescence and early adulthood. At least 1 percent of the population (2.2 million people) suffers from a severe form of it each year, and both men and women are afflicted in equal numbers.

Thanks to new treatments, most who suffer can lead normal lives. Braxton is a good example of this. His medication controls his illness, and he and his wife, who is also mentally ill, monitor themselves closely. Braxton told me that they sit down together every morning and every night to check on each other, making sure they've taken their medication and that they have no signs of "red zones." He is very proud that neither he nor his wife has had an episode now for more than two years. I'm proud of them, too.

The Symptoms of Manic-Depression

Individuals with manic-depressive illness swing from the lows of depression that I've described earlier to the sometimes impossible highs of mania. These acute episodes can alternate with relatively normal times. Braxton Mallard seems to experience more depression as part of his illness, but Margot Kidder tends toward the highs. In an interview she gave when she was nineteen, she said, "I have mood swings that knock over entire cities." But at that time, she had no name for what was bothering her.

"I get more manic than depressed," she told Barbara Walters. "I get really manic. I get way up really fast where your brain starts to go really faster and faster. And then these extraordinarily bizarre leaps in the mind start to happen. . . . You get really revved up. You stop needing to sleep. . . . You stop sleeping, essentially, which makes it much worse."

As do many others with this illness, Kidder has experienced the highs as wonderful. "Sometimes I go soaring up to a place of incredible illumination and wonder," she explained. But then there is the downside. "At other times, the terror of knowing that you are going to a place that is considered mad, and it is mad—let's face it, it is crazy, it is mad—the terror of what is happening to you, the panic that sets in . . ."

At the beginning of the manic phases individuals may feel powerful, full of energy, giddy with excitement, seductive, bubbly, elated, euphoric—in short, pretty terrific. In another interview with a reporter from *People* magazine, Kidder used this description: "When you listen to Beethoven's ninth, you get pleasure, a manic-depressive gets rapture!" But these phases can devolve into much more intense and active periods in which life seems to spin out of control.

According to the American Psychiatric Association, during a manic episode, someone with bipolar illness may:

• Talk too fast, too loud, and without stopping, racing from one idea to the next in rapid succession, but not necessarily logically. This "flight of ideas" can deteriorate into nonsensical communication, thoughts others are unable to follow.

• Be in an exceedingly good mood. In fact, nothing can change this euphoria, not even a tragedy. However, sometimes the mood can turn quickly to irritability, anger, and paranoia (delusions arranged in an orderly sequence, often of persecution, in an otherwise relatively intact personality).

• Move too fast, make too many plans, and behave hyperactively.

• Stop sleeping for days without feeling tired and stop eating.

• Act self-confident and grandiose and express optimism even when the situation doesn't warrant it. Affected individuals may experience delusions of grandeur such as connections with political figures or God, or may believe that the laws of nature do not apply to them.

• Begin many projects at once without the wherewithal to complete them. They may become highly distracted by insignificant details.

• Buy impulsively and excessively or otherwise use poor judgment, such as driving recklessly or making unwise and hasty business investments.

• Engage in promiscuous or unusual sexual behavior.

• Become impatient, irritable, agitated, volatile, violent, and even psychotic when thwarted. Some individuals with manic-depressive illness are sent to prison because their acting-out behavior has led them to break the law.

These manic episodes are nearly always followed by a deep depression. Sometimes this occurs immediately, or a few months can pass before it begins. Then there can be a long interval of normalcy. Severely affected people, however, may have what's called "rapid cycling" bipolar illness, in which the mood swings occur almost continuously.

Suicide can be the result. Margot Kidder admitted to self-mutilation and suicide attempts. "I just always assumed I would kill myself by suicide so I didn't plan for the future," Margot told Barbara Walters. According to the National Institute of

Mental Health, people with untreated manic-depressive illness face up to a 20 percent risk of death by suicide.

Anxiety Disorders

We all feel anxious from time to time—before a big test or presentation, after a fight with our spouse or boss, when we're anticipating a difficult event. A little bit of anxiety keeps us alert, helps us rise to the occasion and meet the challenge head on.

But for people with anxiety disorder, the anxiety escalates until it is incapacitating. It doesn't help them face the world, but rather makes them want to flee it. According to the National Institute of Mental Health anxiety disorders aren't just a case of "nerves." They are illnesses—the most common of all mental illnesses.

There are several types of anxiety disorders, all with their own distinct symptoms. Among the most prevalent are panic disorder, phobias, and obsessive-compulsive disorder (OCD).

Panic Disorder and Phobias

Jerilyn Ross had never had a fear of heights. She loved high places—flying, skiing. Always a risk-taking, adventurous person, she enjoyed going to the top of the Empire State Building and looking out over the edge. Then one day, at the age of twenty-five, while traveling through Europe with an old college roommate, she had an experience that changed her life. "We heard there was a music festival in Salzburg, Austria," she explained, "so we went there. Someone told us about the Café Winkler, which was a really beautiful restaurant and dance place built into a mountain. You take an elevator up to the top and even though you're in a building, you feel as if you're on a mountain.

"There was a verandah overlooking the city. Because of the music festival, the entire city was lit up. It was unbelievably magnificent. The lights were glittering. You could see the castle lights and hear music. I was sitting with my friend, and a guy came over to ask me to dance. We were doing a waltz. I remember thinking, Here I am in this most romantic place, a handsome prince has asked me to dance. We're doing a waltz, and I'm looking out over the city. And then all of a sudden, absolutely out of the blue, I just got knocked by an incredible sense of panic that I was going to jump. I felt like a magnet was pulling me and I was going to go off the edge. I didn't know what was happening. My heart was pounding; I was sweating; I felt like I was about to go crazy.

"Even though this was all going on inside, I remember calmly saying to my dance partner, 'Excuse me, I have to make a phone call.' Who was I going to call? I was in Austria! I left the dance. I had to get out of there. I signaled to my girlfriend that I was in trouble. I remember quietly trying to get through the crowd of tourists to the elevator.

"When we got down to the bottom, I was fine, but I had no idea what had hit me. I knew it was something intense and traumatic, and it felt like an incredibly profound experience. I wasn't depressed, I wasn't suicidal. It made absolutely no sense to me, and I had no idea what was happening. We went back up again, but as soon as I walked out of the elevator, knowing I was up there, the feeling started coming over me again, so we left."

Jerilyn, who has since founded the Anxiety Disorders Association of America, could not shake the feeling. "When I got home to New York, I went to visit my boyfriend. He lived on a high floor. As soon as I stepped out of the elevator, I began to panic, and I told him we had to go downstairs. Within a six-month period, I began to notice that I just couldn't go over the tenth floor in any building. I had no idea why or what was wrong. I was a graduate student in psychology at the time. I spent hours in the library researching my problem. It made no sense. I didn't want to jump. I wasn't suicidal. I wasn't depressed. There was nothing written about it anyplace."

Jerilyn didn't tell anybody about her problem, not even her family, because she felt that she had "deep dark demons" that she didn't understand. "For five years, I lived in Manhattan but could not go above the tenth floor. I continued skiing. During that time, I went to Europe once and skied on a glacier. It never really made any sense to me. It wasn't a fear of heights. It was just a sense of being in a high place where I felt trapped. It was totally irrational. How could I say to someone, 'I'll go skiing with you, dangling from a gondola or a chairlift, but I won't go to a party in your house because you live on the twelfth floor'? What I've learned is that, by definition, a phobia is irrational."

At the age of thirty, Jerilyn read about a small therapy group in New York that was helping people deal with phobias and panic disorder. She quickly joined. "They were very normal people, just like me. There was an attorney, a businessman, and teacher. I realized that I wasn't alone, I wasn't crazy. Other people had it. None of us had dysfunctional lives or families. We all seemed very normal, but we all had this 'thing' that made no sense.

"The way I got help was what I do now with my patients. A therapist literally took me by the hand, and we went one floor at a time past the eighth and ninth floors. My graduation, ten weeks after we had begun therapy, was going to the Gulf + Western Building in New York, which is forty-four stories high, and having a drink on top of the building. I remember looking down at the clouds and thinking that I had won an Olympic medal. I couldn't believe that I was actually doing something that felt so exciting and foreign to me at the same time."

As we have seen from Jerilyn's experience, panic attacks occur suddenly, with no apparent cause, and are terrifying. They usually only last for a few minutes, but when they hit, they make people believe they're dying, or having a heart attack, or just plain losing their minds. Many sufferers end up in the emergency rooms of hospitals.

In panic disorder these attacks keep on happening, and those affected may stay frightened all the time, worrying about when and where the next one will strike. They may even develop phobias (irrational fears) about situations where an attack has occurred—for example, someone who has had a panic attack while driving may be afraid to get behind the wheel again, even to drive to the grocery store. Jerilyn's phobia was fear of high places where she felt trapped.

Millions of people are affected each year, yet until recently these disorders were not taken as serious mental illnesses. "We were considered part of the worried well," Jerilyn explained, "even though many of our people are as incapacitated as others with far more obviously serious mental illnesses. For so long, people were made to feel they were just making it up." Sadly, according to the NIMH, less than 25 percent of those needing treatment for this brain disease ever receive it.

In my foreword to the book Jerilyn wrote about her experiences, *Triumph over Fear,* I explain that people with an anxiety disorder, particularly that 1 percent of the population who suffer from panic disorder, typically see many physicians searching for an explanation for their symptoms. Most often they are labeled "high-strung," "nervous," or as "hypochondriacs," and sent home without obtaining an accurate diagnosis or being told that they have a treatable condition.

When an anxiety disorder is not recognized or appropriately treated, the toll is great, not only for those affected, but also for their families and the community at large. Many people with panic disorder, for instance, have markedly constrained lifestyles because of fear of traveling any distance from home, which often leaves them unable to fulfill family and career responsibilities and social obligations. In addition, one third of people with anxiety disorders abuse alcohol, which brings an additional and separate set of problems. Many also suffer from depression at the same time.

Thanks to national public and professional education programs including those spearheaded by Jerilyn's organization, the Anxiety Disorders Association of America, and to NIMH, these diseases are now more frequently and accurately diagnosed by the medical community.

The Symptoms of Panic Disorder and Phobias

The typical symptoms of anxiety disorders can include:

- Dizziness, sweating, cold flashes, shakiness, trembling, and/or faintness
- Nausea or abdominal distress
- Tightness in the chest, racing or pounding heartbeat
- Difficulty breathing, shortness of breath, and choking
- Terror—a sense that something unimaginably horrible is about to occur and one is powerless to prevent it
- Fear of losing control and doing something embarrassing
- Fear of dying
- Feelings of unreality

Persistent worry about having another attack and changes in behavior to avoid it are also part of this illness. People with anxiety disorders can sometimes become so incapacitated, their lives so restricted, that they avoid normal, everyday activities such as grocery shopping or driving. Some even become prisoners of their own homes, literally for years. This type of panic disorder is called agoraphobia.

About a third of those with panic disorder develop agoraphobia. According to the APA, about two thirds of sufferers are women. This may be due only to the fact that women are more likely to seek treatment. Some experts hypothesize that male sufferers medicate themselves with alcohol or by abusing drugs.

Panic disorder is real and can be disabling, but it can be treated effectively. Also, early treatment can often stop the progression to agoraphobia. People who have panic attacks should be taken seriously. Trying to reassure them with expressions such as "It's nothing serious," "It's all in your head," or "It's nothing to worry about" may be harmful and keep them from seeking help.

Obsessive-Compulsive Disorder (OCD)

Jeffrey M. Schwartz, a research psychiatrist at the University of California, Los Angeles, has treated more than a thousand patients with OCD. He characterizes the disorder as "brain lock." In his book of the same name, he writes, "We call this problem 'brain lock' because four key structures of the brain become locked together, and the brain starts sending false messages that the person cannot readily recognize as false."

Dr. Schwartz explains that victims of OCD engage in bizarre and self-destructive behaviors in order to prevent some imagined catastrophe. "But there is no realistic connection between the behaviors and the catastrophes they so fear." Sufferers of this illness, for example, may take literally the childhood ditty "Step on a crack, break your mother's back."

The Symptoms of Obsessive-Compulsive Disorder

People with OCD are plagued by:

Obsessions: intrusive and distressing thoughts that can include:

- Unwarranted fears about the family's safety, contamination, or neatness or symmetry
- Repetitive rituals and questions for no logical reason
- Unfounded fears about not paying bills or doing routine tasks
- Excessive concerns about blasphemous thoughts or morality
- Fear of having hurt someone or of acting out violent thoughts

Compulsions: repeated behaviors in which they engage to rid themselves of the fears that their obsessive thoughts create:

- Constant washing
- Counting
- Checking of appliances or door locks
- Hoarding of useless articles
- Adjustment of household items to preserve symmetry
- Checking and rechecking of bank balances
- The need to touch or tap certain objects repeatedly or for a ritualized number of times

"When the brain gets stuck," Schwartz explains, "it may tell you, 'You must wash your hands again,' and you'll wash, even though there is no real reason to do so." Unfortunately, once people give in to these irresistible urges, their compulsions become even stronger. "The person with OCD," Schwartz writes, "washes and washes, even though it causes him great pain and gives him no pleasure. . . . Those with OCD realize how inappropriate their behavior is, are ashamed and embarrassed by it, and are in the truest sense desperate to change their behavior."

Although anxiety disorders such as these can be disabling, they are highly responsive to treatment. As Jerilyn Ross explained, "The good news and the message I always want to get out is that these disorders are real, serious, and they're treatable. We can successfully treat up to 90 percent of people with these disorders."

❧

In this chapter, I have laid out the major characteristics of the most prevalent mental illnesses and illustrated these through the personal stories of men and women who have been willing to share their pains and triumphs with us. They have done so in the belief that their experiences will help others better understand their own illnesses and have hope about successful treatment. In subsequent chapters, we will look at the amazing developments in brain research and treatment that are now helping to relieve so many people of their suffering. But first, I'd like to take a further look at why we call mental illnesses "equal opportunity" problems.

Chapter 3

An Equal Opportunity Problem

Did you know that Dick Cavett, Mike Wallace, and Art Buchwald have all suffered from depression? The *Today* show weatherman, Willard Scott, has overcome a panic disorder. And Patty Duke wrote a memoir about her experiences with manic-depression.

One of the striking aspects of mental illnesses is that they know no boundaries. People of all groups, no matter where they live or what their wealth, race, or age might be, suffer from these conditions—although certain illnesses may affect some groups more than others.

Different people have different ways of dealing with mental problems. Some, in a misguided effort to medicate themselves, turn to illicit drugs and alcohol. For those living in poverty or for the working poor who have no health insurance, care is limited. Illiteracy, ignorance, or cultural beliefs about the mind and body may stand in the way of others receiving treatment. Children must depend on adults to recognize their condition and seek therapy, and elderly citizens may have to depend on their children. Yet with awareness, education, and proper treatment, much can be done today to alleviate this needless suffering.

Do Men or Women Suffer More?

Certain mental illnesses—depression and anxiety disorders, in particular—seem to strike women twice as frequently as men, while others such as bipolar illness and schizophrenia occur with relatively equal frequency in the two genders (see appendix B). Much has been written in an attempt to explain this, particularly in the case of depression.

Why are women twice as likely to suffer from depression as men? Researchers have theorized that:

• Women are more likely to seek help, and therefore are more apt to be counted in surveys.

• Hormonal and other biological differences between men and women (which contribute to premenstrual syndrome, postpartum depression, and the emotional impact of infertility and miscarriage) may foster depressed moods.

• Some speculate that more women are depressed than men "due to their experience being female in our contemporary culture."[1] Social factors including less favorable job and economic opportunities and differing social roles, positions, and upbringing could all be contributing factors.

• Women and children constitute 75 percent of the people living in poverty in the United States. Poverty has been identified as a "pathway to depression."[2]

• Victimization, sexual or physical abuse in childhood or adulthood, conditions that appear to affect more women than men, and the resulting post-traumatic stress disorder (nightmares, flashbacks, anxiety) could trigger depression.

• Marriage and children have been related to a higher incidence of depression in women—the more children in the family, the higher the rate of occurrence.

Men commit suicide four times as often as women do. It has been suggested that this reflects differences in the way men and women cope (or fail to cope) with depression. Some psychologists have found that when things go badly in women's lives, they tend to blame themselves, while men in similar situations tend to point the finger outwardly.[3] Terrence Real, a therapist who has written a book on male depression entitled *I Don't Want to Talk About It,* explains, "This is one major reason depressed men may strike out at their wives, their children, their co-workers. And if they can't, they'll find addictions to soothe the pain, self-medicating with sex, gambling, booze."[4]

Alcohol, though ultimately a depressant, can temporarily improve one's mood and ease depressive symptoms such as loss of appetite, low energy, and insomnia. Cocaine and many other illicit drugs are mood elevators and will also temporarily alleviate signs of depression.

A recent survey of the Amish, who almost never drink or abuse drugs, found that men and women in that unique community have identical rates of major depression and bipolar illness. These results suggest that the incidence of depressive disorders may be the same in men and women, but that men's different coping mechanisms, including drinking and drug use, simply mask the symptoms.[5]

The same may be true of anxiety disorders, since they too are reported in twice as many women as men. Studies show that 10 to 20 percent of people with social phobias (extreme shyness in the presence of others) use alcohol to alleviate their anxiety. And a third of alcoholics report a history of panic disorder or social phobia before they started drinking. In scientific terms, the occurrence of any two or more mental illnesses or mental illness and substance abuse at the same time is called dual diagnosis or comorbidity.[6]

Dual Diagnosis and Comorbidity

The author William Styron describes the relationship between his alcoholism and the onset of depression in his memoir *Darkness Visible*. At one point in his life he found that alcohol, formerly his "great ally," suddenly sickened him. "I could no longer drink," he wrote. "It was as if my body had risen up in protest, along with my mind, and had conspired to reject this daily mood bath which it had so long welcomed. . . . Suddenly vanished, the great ally which for so long had kept my demons at bay was no longer there to prevent those demons from beginning to swarm through the subconscious, and I was emotionally naked, vulnerable as I had never been before. . . . There were also dreadful, pouncing seizures of anxiety."[7]

Styron's description is well founded. Drugs of abuse may precipitate or exacerbate mental illness; by the same token, self-medication for mental illness may result in drug abuse or addiction. It is a vicious cycle. Individuals with untreated mental disorders are at much greater risk for substance abuse than those who are not ill.[8]

Consider Larry Fricks, the head of consumer relations at the Georgia Division of Mental Health in Atlanta. Before his bipolar illness was diagnosed and treated, he had used alcohol to mute the highs of the manic phases and cocaine to bring him up when he was depressed.[9] My neighbor Braxton Mallard had abused Valium in his attempts to regulate his moods, and actress Margot Kidder tried to hide her symptoms with alcohol and drugs. Ironically, as Ms. Kidder explained, it seems to be more socially acceptable to admit to a substance abuse problem than a mental illness.

As one writer so aptly put it, "Like a stealth submarine, a mood or personality disorder often lurks undetected beneath an ocean of alcohol or drug abuse."[10]

Children Have Mental Illness Too

For many years, psychiatrists did not believe that children could suffer from mental illnesses—that their minds were not developed enough to experience serious mental or emotional problems. But childhood mental illnesses are real and depression, for example, can occur in children as young as seven or eight years old. Other mental illnesses may show their first signs even earlier. We don't know all the causes of mental health problems in young people, but we do know that biology and environment can both be involved, as with all mental illnesses.

While scientists are seeking the biological causes, we know of many environmental factors that can put children at risk. Among them are exposure to violence, abuse, neglect, lead poisoning, or loss of loved ones through death, divorce, or broken relationships. Other factors include rejection because of race, religion, or poverty.

Studies suggest that about one in five young Americans suffers from mental disorders; of these, 7.5 million children are thought to be severely impaired.[11] Tragically, very few of those affected receive treatment. Too often their problems are not recognized by parents, teachers, or doctors. Yet untreated children may not simply "outgrow" their difficulties; they may instead develop into seriously mentally ill adults.

Anxiety disorders, for example, double the risk of later substance abuse, and untreated depression in children and preteens can lead to suicidal behavior. Suicide is the third leading cause of death among people aged fifteen to twenty-four and the fourth leading cause of death for youngsters ten to fourteen years of age.

The good news is that depression in children and adolescents is amenable to treatment with new, highly effective medications. Because these medications are so effective, they are already being widely prescribed even though Food and Drug Administration guidelines for young people have not yet been fully established. (In 1996, more than half a million children and adolescents received a prescription for Paxil, Zoloft, or Prozac to treat depression and anxiety disorders.[12]) Medications, however, are not the only treatment for depression or other mental disorders in children. Individual and family therapy and, for those with serious mental disturbances, comprehensive services can be effective.

The case of Matthew Stauffer illustrates the mental disorder that is most common in children: *attention deficit hyperactivity disorder* (ADHD), also called *attention deficit disorder* (ADD).[13] Parents and teachers struggle with this hyperactive behavior when a child is affected.

Matthew's mother, as reported in *USA Today,* first noticed the change in her son the summer he turned seven.[14] He would write on the floor of his bedroom and the walls of the den with crayon. There would be angry outbursts, "very juvenile behavior," his mother said.

When school started, things got worse. Matthew's behavior in class became disruptive; he could not concentrate long enough to listen to instructions. Then he would be too embarrassed to ask the teacher to repeat them, so he would act like a class clown to try to get attention, bothering other students to hide his own inability to concentrate. His self-esteem sank to the point where any rebuke or correction would make him feel terrible about himself. The teacher was understandably upset.

It was November before the Stauffers took Matthew to a psychologist for tests. That's when they learned that their son had ADHD, which is six to nine times more common in boys than in girls. Its symptoms include extreme fidgeting, distraction (short attention span, tendency to be easily diverted by things others ignore), and impulsivity (not stopping to think before acting).[15]

Although ADHD cannot be cured, thousands of youngsters have been helped to focus on their schoolwork and better manage their social relations with a combination of educational therapy, family therapy, behavior modification, and/or medication. Matthew Stauffer is one who has improved on Ritalin, which he calls his "thinking pills."

Anxiety disorders are also quite common among children,[16] and the problem can start at a very early age. Separation disorder (extreme fear of leaving home and parents) can begin at an average age of eight, and overanxious disorders (school avoidance and extreme fear of strangers) can first appear at about ten years of age. The onset of panic disorder in children reaches its peak in the sixth or seventh grade.

More than one of these anxiety disorders can occur in children at the same time; they can also occur in combination with other disorders such as depression. Evidence also indicates that they may be enduring. According to Jerilyn Ross, who has suffered from panic disorder and phobia, "Many patients first diagnosed with panic disorder in adulthood recall symptoms during childhood."

Children who wake up many times during the night or make unusually ritualized demands and try to dictate the lives of other family members may be suffering from obsessive-compulsive disorder. A child with this disorder can wreak havoc on a family. UCLA research psychiatrist Jeffrey M. Schwartz explains in his book *Brain Lock* that parents become engaged in this behavior because they have heaped guilt upon themselves, "convinced that they are responsible for the child having this awful illness." Clearly they are not.

Children's conduct disorders may begin in the preschool years but do not become fully apparent until later childhood or adolescence. Affected children persistently engage in antisocial behaviors such as aggression, theft, fire setting, and vandalism. They initiate fights and can be physically cruel to people and animals. Often these youngsters have a history of truancy from school and episodes of running away from home.

Children may also suffer from *Tourette's syndrome,* in which they are plagued by volleys of tics, squeaks, growls, and curse words they cannot suppress; *autism,* a pervasive developmental disorder in which they have been described as being "locked in a strange and speechless world almost no one can penetrate"; and *eating disorders,* which are especially common among adolescent girls, and include excessive dieting, binge eating, laxative abuse, and purging.

Childhood schizophrenia was once thought to be a form of autism, but MRI scans (brain imaging techniques that show the brain in action) show some of the same abnormalities found in adults with the disease.[17] Sadly, childhood schizophrenia can be a more harmful disorder, because damage to brain development begins so early.

All of these problems cause misery for children and their families, and a decade ago the outlook for these children was bleak. They might have been dismissed as just "moody teenagers" or "bad children." Today, thanks to research, many of these seriously ill young people can, with treatment, lead normal lives largely free of illness. But early intervention is a must. When we delay, we run the risk of our children growing into adults with full-blown disabilities.

Mental Illness and the Elderly

How often have we heard it said of an elderly friend, neighbor, or relative, "Of course Nancy is depressed. It's normal for a widow to be depressed." Or, "Jack will be okay. Give him a couple of months. Everyone gets down after a heart attack." A recent Harris poll commissioned by the Geriatric Psychiatry Alliance found that 93 percent of Americans believe depression is a "normal" and inevitable reaction to disease and not an illness in itself.

The truth is, no matter what one's age or situation, depression is not "normal." It is an illness that can be treated effectively. As Jimmy and I explained in our book *Everything to Gain: Making the Most of the Rest of Your Life,* most older Americans are not depressed. They cope well and lead remarkably active, productive lives. Even among those who must endure medical illness, financial reverses, and personal loss, many remain mentally healthy. Although multiple forms of mental disorders can begin late in life, they are not an inevitable part of the aging process.

And yet, of the 32 million Americans over age sixty-five, an estimated four million suffer from dementing disorders, including Alzheimer's disease; nearly 5 million experience serious symptoms of depression; and 1 million suffer from major depression. In addition, many elderly people experience anxiety, stress, sleep disorders, loneliness, social isolation, fear of abandonment, and abuse.

Depression is the most common disorder and the leading cause of suicide among the elderly. Although 13 percent of the U.S. population is over age sixty-five, this age group accounts for 20 percent of all suicides. Men who are seventy-five years or older have the highest suicide rate of any age group, worldwide.[18] And 90 percent of those who commit suicide have at least one diagnosable mental or substance abuse disorder.

What can account for these disproportionately high numbers among the elderly? Many are not getting needed psychiatric services—either because they or their families do not recognize and/or report their symptoms to their physician or because medical professionals fail to recognize the problem.[19]

Apathy or vague physical complaints can also mask depressive symptoms. Studies have shown that three quarters of elderly men who committed suicide saw their doctor in the month before they killed themselves, but practically none had consulted mental health professionals and very few had received appropriate treatment.

Depression can also be dangerous for the elderly because it aggravates other medical conditions. Studies show it significantly increases the rate of stroke and the risk of heart attack, hip fracture, and severe infection. There is some debate in scientific circles as to which comes first—the mental illness or the medical condition. In the case of heart disease, for example, one group attributes heart disease to biochemical changes in the brain (the secretion of stress hormones) in those who are depressed, causing erratic heartbeats and increased cholesterol levels. The other group believes that those who are depressed are less likely to be vigilant about their diet, medication schedule, or the management of high blood pressure, thereby predisposing themselves to heart attacks.[20]

Mental or emotional disorders in elderly citizens can also be caused or aggravated by physical illnesses or their treatments. Drug reactions, unrecognized endocrine problems (low thyroid function, for example), pain from osteoporosis or arthritis, and even undiagnosed hearing or visual impairment can account for about half of the elderly patients seen in mental health clinics and hospitals. Depression and anxiety disorders can also accompany cancer, insomnia, diabetes, strokes, influenza, post-surgical confusion, and Parkinson's disease.

Depression among the elderly is often misdiagnosed. In some cases, the confusion and memory loss associated with it can be mistaken for Alzheimer's disease or "senility." If depression is truly the cause of these symptoms, it can be reversed with proper treatment. Alzheimer's, the slow deterioration of brain function eventually leading to death, will not improve with therapy, but treatment can enhance an Alzheimer's sufferer's quality of life and coping skills.

Because depression can impair one's judgment, the safest course of action is to seek medical care from a professional trained in geriatric psychiatry, as Eunice McKinnery did.[21]

"I just wanted to lie down, and I didn't want to be bothered with anyone," Eunice recalled. "I had a bad feeling." But her family realized that her lethargy and lack of appetite were a problem and took her to the geriatric psychiatry wing at Wills Hospital in Philadelphia. Within a few weeks she was back in her apartment, "feeling fantastic," Eunice said.

Unfortunately, many elderly are not so lucky. Harry Nance, sixty-six, was misdiagnosed for decades. He finally got help when "I did something that old hill folks don't like to do." He asked for food stamps. When he did, a perceptive caseworker told him she would get food stamps for him if he saw someone for treatment. He did. His depression was stabilized, and he was able to return to his original profession.

I fully agree with Ira R. Katz, past president of the Geriatric Psychiatric Alliance, who testified before Congress, "We have an optimistic view of the aging process and a conviction that older people have an impressive ability to lead pleasurable and meaningful lives in spite of the stresses of aging and medical illness, if, but only if, their depression is recognized and treated."[22]

Mental Illness Among Ethnic Groups—No Group Is Immune

For many reasons, certain issues are more difficult to deal with in particular groups.

Consider the question of suicide among young people, which has been strongly linked to mental illness and also to substance abuse. Kenya Napper Bello is a woman with a mission— a mission born of tragedy. In November of 1994, a scant six months after her marriage to Razak, a twenty-seven-year-old executive at the Coca-Cola Company and a graduate student at Johns Hopkins University's School of Advanced International Studies, Razak took his life by jumping from a tall building in downtown Atlanta.

Zac, as Kenya calls her late husband, suffered from manic-depressive illness, but he was too proud to take his medication. He believed that with an intelligent mind, healthy eating habits, and regular exercise, he could control this biochemical brain disease. An African-American, he feared the stigma would jeopardize his hard-won accomplishments and his employment. In the end, however, the disordered behavior that characterized his manic phases caused him to lose his job. And that loss, coupled with a debilitating depression that interfered with his ability to study, left him feeling hopeless and in despair.

Kenya wrote about her experiences in the newsletter of Free Mind Generation, the organization she founded to help combat the stigma associated with suicide and mental illness in the black community. "I believed with a loving wife, supportive family and friends, a man of his strong character would get through this period. This thinking inevitably proved naïve and fatal. Razak needed more than a strong will and a loving hand. He needed medical treatment."[23]

Razak Bello's untimely death is part of a growing trend within the African-American community. While it had always been assumed that "black men don't commit suicide," today the suicide rate among young black males is soaring. According to a 1996 study by the Centers for Disease Control (CDC), it is up

63 percent from 1980 in men between the ages of fifteen and twenty-four, and 300 percent in boys aged ten to fourteen.[24]

Many reasons have been advanced for this increase, including the ready availability of firearms; the persistence of racial discrimination in the workplace; the poverty, hopelessness, and high stress that urban youth experience; the breakdown of traditional black families and the waning influence of the church; substance abuse; and living with a history of violence.

The statistics for suicide, historically low for African-Americans when compared with whites, may have been skewed by what social scientists call "victim-precipitated homicides"—suicides in which someone else does the killing. A victim may purposely put himself in harm's way—waving a gun, for example, in the faces of rival gang members—because it is more socially acceptable to be killed by others than to kill oneself. Single car accidents, drug overdoses, and accidental shootings in front of friends may not be counted as suicides, even if they are.

"Some commit suicide by their own hands; others position themselves in the line of fire," Kenya Bello explained. "Anyone who chooses this way out is most often protesting an unbearable pain, a pain rooted in hopelessness. I get letters from African-American men in prison. Their situations were so difficult, they didn't care about life. They didn't care if they hurt themselves or others."

Suicides among Hispanic youth take a different course. Although Hispanic teenagers have relatively low suicide death rates, they are nearly twice as likely to have made a suicide attempt as their African-American and non-Hispanic white classmates.[25] They are also more likely to harbor serious suicidal thoughts. In a recent CDC study, 25 percent of Hispanic high school girls reported making specific suicide plans in the previous year, compared with 15.5 percent of their black peers.

Why should this population attempt suicide so frequently? Perhaps those who are children of immigrant parents have trouble adjusting to a new culture. Perhaps their families fled strife and civil turmoil. Studies show that a high proportion of immigrant children are diagnosed with mental illnesses including anxiety disorders, depression, and post-traumatic stress disorder. Perhaps also, since there are still relatively few Spanish-speaking mental health professionals or low-cost mental health services in Hispanic communities, few have access to care. It is a fact that the Hispanic-American community has the largest percentage of uninsured youth in the nation.

If culturally appropriate services were available and affordable, perhaps the number of suicide attempts—and the despair, anxiety, and depression that they bespeak—would be greatly reduced.

This issue is not as clear in the Asian-American community, especially among recent immigrants. Mental illnesses are highly stigmatized in some Southeast Asian cultures. Having a family member with a mental disorder can affect one's social status and ability to marry; as a result, family members may consider it their responsibility to care for a mentally ill relative at home, turning to a mental health agency only when in dire need.

All of these ethnic issues point to the importance of understanding the impact of one's culture on mental health. Our culture helps to determine how we define mental illness and whether we seek treatment.

The Impact of Culture

When the President's Commission on Mental Health was conducting public hearings around the country in 1978, I remember meeting a Haitian immigrant living in Phoenix who had gone to a therapist to confess her fear that her husband's ex-wife had put a hex on her! The therapist diagnosed her as paranoid and prescribed Thorazine, a powerful anti-psychotic medication. Yet further exploration of her case by a bicultural therapist revealed that she was not paranoid at all, and that hers was a common dilemma in her culture.

In city after city, we heard similar tales of misunderstanding and discrimination from African-Americans, Hispanic-Americans, Native Americans, and Asian-Americans who faced difficulties in obtaining culturally appropriate services.

Everyone in the world belongs to a culture. Our culture affects how we interpret our environment and our relationships. The official handbook of illnesses that mental health professionals rely upon for diagnosis, *The Diagnostic and Statistical Manual of Mental Disorders (DSM-IV™),* has finally begun to address these cultural issues.[26] For example, it now lists a set of symptoms for the Malaysian problem called *amok,* a belief in possession by a spirit that causes shouting, laughing, and head-banging but is not considered abnormal in that society.

Recognizing and understanding cultural differences is important because of the danger of misdiagnosis and inappropriate treatment. If a patient and therapist do not speak the same language or if they come from different ethnic backgrounds, culturally associated nuances can be missed. What may look like a delusion or hallucination to a therapist in one society, in another society may be a normal, culturally based reaction. In cultures in which the needs of the individual are secondary to those of the family, as in Asian communities, individual therapy may seem threatening or inappropriate. Sometimes, individuals may lack trust in the therapists because of prior negative experiences or simply because in their cultures, speaking with outsiders about personal problems is taboo.

Child-rearing practices vary from culture to culture. Peruvian Inca children, for instance, are taught to be reserved and quiet, whereas children coming from Caribbean cultures can be more expressive and sociable. Since shame plays a formidable role in shaping behavior and maintaining traditions in many Asian cultures, failure and loss of face can disturb an Asian-American individual in ways that other Americans may not understand. African-American families may be as diverse as any other ethnic group in our nation, but all must cope with threatened, perceived, and/or actual racism and its consequences to mental health.

In *The New York Times,* science writer Daniel Goleman reported on a case in which a culturally sensitive approach made all the difference. After an uncle with whom she was particularly close died suddenly in Ecuador, a seemingly psychotic New York woman, listless and disorganized, complained to her family, "My soul is not with me anymore—I can't do anything." Fortunately, at the psychiatric hospital to which she was taken, a therapist recognized that she was suffering from a Latin American problem called *susto,* or loss of the soul with the death of a loved one. While we might have viewed her state as depression, the patient felt as if her soul had departed with her uncle.

Treatment for her was brief, and simply involved several individual and family therapy sessions coupled with a Hispanic mourning ritual. Soon her symptoms were gone, and she returned to her normal level of functioning.

For proper diagnosis and treatment, individuals must be understood within their cultural context.

The Homeless and Mental Illness

Tim was familiar with the "cat holes" in Atlanta, vacant houses he could find to sleep in at night. He had few possessions, which he usually carried around with him. If he left anything at the cat hole during the day, it was almost surely gone when he returned at night. He was a young man, tall, slender, with a head full of dark, curly hair. Unkempt from the exposure and suffering from asthma, Tim had been homeless for about a year and a half. Most of the time he kept to himself on the streets, not sharing his burdens with anyone.

Most of us will never be forced to endure the fear, despair, and helplessness that are so much a part of homelessness. But hundreds of thousands of our fellow Americans do. Some arrive at this point because of chronic mental illness. Tim suffers from major depression.

He came to live at O'Hern House in March 1997. Part of Project Interconnections, a program in Atlanta that I have been involved with for many years, O'Hern House is a "low impact" residence especially designed for severely mentally ill people who don't want to come off the streets. Because many have had prior negative experiences in institutions, they trust no one. O'Hern House tries to address the residents' needs and still let them retain their independence. New residents are not required to bathe or check in and out. They can even sleep on the floor if they wish. The low demands make it easier for them to accept shelter and gain confidence in the staff, who in turn can then help them begin treatment.

I talked with Tim recently at O'Hern House about his illness and his experiences. He told me that looking back he thought he had dealt with depression ever since childhood. He said his early family life was "weird." There was no discipline in his home. "Everything was permissible." He began to drink when he was only about ten years old. His brothers and sisters said it was okay. He also experimented with drugs at this very early age. That was okay, too. It was even okay not to go to school.

71

Tim never felt that he got any support from his family; rather, he always felt detached from them—even ostracized. He had to make adult decisions as a child: what he could and couldn't do. When he was about thirteen, he began staying away from home, coming in very late in the evenings. No one cared.

Very early, he had made the right decision about school, attending and graduating from high school. Continuing his education, he became a certified medical assistant and worked in the health care field for fourteen years.

Tim told me that he certainly couldn't call himself stable during this period, but he was functional. Often despondent, though, he had trouble holding down a job, moving from one to another.

Then in 1987, Tim was diagnosed as HIV-positive. For the next five years, he carried this burden alone. He didn't share it with his family or friends. For a while after the diagnosis, he tried to keep working, but he couldn't concentrate on what he was doing. Thus began the downward spiral that left him sleeping in cat holes and on the streets. Lonely, isolated, and feeling utterly helpless, he became suicidal, obsessed with dying—not eating, not sleeping, and abusing drugs in an effort to escape his misery.

"By 1993," he said, "I had gone as far as I could go trying to deal with the diagnosis of terminal illness alone. One day I found myself in a shopping mall, confused and disoriented. A policeman took me to the hospital, where for the first time I was officially diagnosed with clinical depression and given medication."

Once out and back on the streets, he took his medication for a while. "Then," he said, "when I would feel good, I would stop taking my medicine and be back in the hospital before I knew it." Over the next few years he was in and out of hospitals, being treated for depression and substance abuse.

In early 1997, while in an Atlanta hospital, it was so obvious that he needed more help in dealing with his problems that he was referred to our program, Project Interconnections. That is how he got to O'Hern House.

"I am blessed," Tim says. "I now have a safe and secure environment. I know I am not going to be harmed. I take my medication and I know there is a support system here for me twenty-four hours a day."

The O'Hern House staff is optimistic about Tim's slow, steady recovery. He says it is a daily process for him, having to deal with his terminal illness, though he still has had no sick days from it.

Tim is now working as a work opportunity employee at O'Hern House. He is coeditor of the program's newsletter and is running for office in the tenants' association. Just before Christmas, he helped organize a coat and clothing drive, which was widely publicized in the city, and clothes are "still coming in from everywhere. We're planning on opening a clothes closet," he said, "so when people come in with no clothes we will have some for them." His latest venture is organizing a gospel choir, hoping to bring happiness into some lives.

"The Lord is going to see me through this," Tim says. "If it can't be with a physical healing, then it can be a spiritual healing. While I can, I want to give back."

Tim's story offers us hope and insight. Hope, because we see that it is possible for someone who has been chronically mentally ill, destitute, and on the streets to find a haven and the chance for recovery from the mental illness. Insight, because it reminds us that those who are mentally ill and homeless are people, after all, with families and histories and potential. So often we lose sight of the fact that beneath their tattered clothes, unruly appearance, and bizarre behavior these are individuals who are suffering mentally and often physically as well.[27]

Although it is difficult to estimate accurately the number of people who are homeless in our nation,[28] in 1996 the National Law Center on Homelessness and Poverty put the figure at about 700,000. The National Institute of Mental Health estimates that about one third of these are severely and persistently mentally ill, though some studies indicate that the figure is much higher.[29]

A. M. Rosenthal, after walking past several destitute mentally ill people on the way to his office one morning, posed the question in a *New York Times* editorial: "How did we get to this point, where Americans calmly accept the fact that we cannot deal decently with scores of thousands of destitute Americans that suffer so desperately in their minds that they cry their pain in the streets, where we send them to live? When and why did this country accept madness on the streets as part of the city scenery, turn its back on deeply disturbed [individuals] . . . ?"[30]

It has become routine to blame the large numbers of homeless mentally ill individuals on deinstitutionalization, which did help create the crisis. As Dr. E. Fuller Torrey, research psychiatrist at the Neuroscience Center of NIMH, writes in his book *Out of the Shadows,* "For a substantial minority . . . deinstitutionalization has been a psychiatric *Titanic.*" It is important, however, not to overestimate the impact of that policy. Most of those patients were released in the 1960s and 1970s when states were making the move from large institutions to community-based care. The astonishing increases that we have sadly become accustomed to did not occur until later. While it is still unclear why some mentally ill people become homeless when most do not, the National Coalition for the Homeless reminds us that housing and income subsidies—the safety net for those living on the margins of society—were slashed dramatically during the 1980s.

Low-income people have a hard time obtaining housing. Adding to this are the current problems in the health care system. Millions of Americans have no health care insurance. Even for those who do, the costs of hospitalization for mental illnesses far surpass what insurance companies will pay.

Substance abuse is another factor. Unfortunately, even when these individuals can get their drug or alcohol problems under control by enrolling in a treatment program, often they are discharged back to the streets or shelters, making relapse almost inevitable.

The sad result of this complex set of circumstances is the present situation. And once on the streets, those who suffer have great difficulty obtaining access to mental health treatment, medical care, case management, substance abuse treatment, supportive housing, employment, and even their SSI benefits.

In today's environment of budget cuts, the prospects for any successful effort to bring an end to this devastating problem are not bright. Federal, state, and local programs fall far short. As A. M. Rosenthal says, "If we won't put up the taxes—yes, taxes . . ." But the price we pay for not putting up taxes to care for those who suffer this indignity is enormous. We pay through lost lives, lost productivity; we pay through the welfare system, the housing, health care, and criminal justice systems. And this does not include the cost in terms of misery and suffering for those affected and for their families, which is immeasurable.

So what can be done about the problem? We must continue to lobby for better services. And we can join the growing number of concerned and caring citizens, working through both public and private organizations, who are struggling to provide essential resources in their communities.

Project Interconnections in Atlanta is one example of what can be done all across the country. The program, organized by private citizens to help provide housing for mentally ill people on the streets, now serves 160 at three sites. O'Hern House, where Tim lives, is one of them. Plans are under way to provide for 250 units by the year 2000, and a fourth site is already under construction. While O'Hern House is the only "low impact" facility, all provide independent living, designed for people who, with some supervision, are able to work and live productive lives.

On-site support services for the residents of these facilities are provided primarily by the state, with some federal help through rent subsidies. We have been blessed in Atlanta by the cooperation from the state government and by the exceptional support from the community in fund-raising and in volunteer efforts.

Portals, in Los Angeles, is another innovative residential program for homeless mentally ill people. It is funded by private donations, public funds such as grants from the U.S. Department of Housing and Urban Development, and income that the residents themselves generate from the small gourmet cookie, janitorial, and printing businesses they operate within the framework of the organization.

Victor Angeles, a slender man of forty-one, was homeless, suffering from schizophrenia and substance abuse. Portals changed his life. "It's almost a miracle," he said about his recovery.

After repeated hospitalizations, failed attempts at Alcoholics Anonymous programs, and misguided forays into spiritualism, he found his way to Portals, where he received medication and job training. Soon he became a reporter for the program's daily bulletin. He enrolled in a local community college and took a course in computer-aided drafting. When a job became available on the Portals staff as a trainee to assist a case manager, he jumped at the opportunity. Now Victor helps other residents reach their goals.

"It's very rewarding for me and good for my soul," Victor explained. "I know what the others are going through, and I see myself in their struggles coping with mental illness. . . . My past experiences including my years of addiction, mental illness, and homelessness make me understand human suffering. . . . Those years have prepared me.

"And people look at me differently now. I get compliments. 'You should be proud,' they say. 'You've come a long way.' But I know I couldn't have done it by myself. I tried. God knows I tried. But it was impossible, just impossible by myself."

Chapter 4

When Someone You Love Has a Mental Illness: Seeking Treatment

Susie, a young woman who was a college friend of my son, called one day to ask for my help. Her husband, Bob, was mentally ill, and she was at her wits' end, not knowing where to go or what to do anymore. When I began writing this book, she offered to share her painful memories of that time, in the hope that her experience would help someone else.

Shortly after Susie and Bob were married, Bob started studying accounting. At first they were happy, but during his senior year, Bob seemed overloaded with work, retreating into books. On the Sunday morning he was to graduate, with the CPA exam still looming ahead, he came to Susie and said, "I can't go. I have a brain tumor." He began to cry.

Something was obviously wrong. Not knowing what to do, Susie turned to her minister. Unfortunately, he took her concerns about Bob more seriously than he took Bob's problems. When she told him what had happened, his first question was, "What do you have against men crying?" Bob was sitting there, reticent. It was a delicate situation. She couldn't say the things she wanted to say, and the minister kept questioning her motives. It was humiliating.

Bob's condition grew worse. He became self-destructive, and one day he kept punching the wall until his fist bled. Terrified, Susie couldn't get him to stop. She finally took all the pots and pans out of the cabinet and dropped them on the kitchen floor. The noise got his attention.

Throughout the summer, he continued to beat on things or hit himself so hard with objects that occasionally he wound up in the hospital. Susie was at a loss to know what to do. When she suggested he see a psychiatrist, Bob refused; he even refused to see the family doctor. Susie talked with his parents, but his father, a local business executive, believed that one should "pull yourself up by your bootstraps." Eventually, though, after seeing him at his worst on several occasions, his father recommended a psychiatrist, and Bob went to the doctor.

But it was still downhill. The psychiatrist, conscious of the family's social status, didn't want to admit that Bob had a serious mental illness. He prescribed medication and told him he was going to be all right. Of course, he was not.

Bob was convinced that he was dying of a serious illness. He would ask Susie, "Do you see the spots on my arm?" When she would say that she couldn't, he would grow belligerent. At times he seemed to be in a trance that would last for hours; if interrupted, he became violent.

They spent all their meager savings that fall, going from one doctor to another. None were helpful. One physician, ignoring Susie's pleas, accused them of coming with a "made-up" illness. He proceeded to give her fatherly advice, telling her that she should just slow down for a while!

"It was the most intense isolation one could ever imagine," Susie said. She knew of no resources. She couldn't talk to anyone, including Bob's family; they didn't want to hear. The neighbors knew something was wrong because they saw an ambulance arrive several times, but they never mentioned it. Sometimes, though, Susie would come home and find that her lawn had been mowed.

Bob attempted suicide three times before he finally got help. After the third try, while he was still in the hospital, Susie called me in desperation. I suggested she contact her local affiliate of the National Alliance for the Mentally Ill, because the NAMI organizations are made up of family members of people with mental illness. Many of them have had experiences similar to hers. She found the number listed in the telephone book and called immediately. They were very helpful, telling her what to say to the doctor and giving her many questions to ask. They also gave her the names of support groups and people who had experienced similar problems.

When she got back to Bob's room after making the telephone calls, she saw to her dismay that the doctor was preparing to send him home, saying, "He's just not sick." Bob had charmed them all.

"Don't!" she cried. And this time his parents, too, admitted that he needed help. Bob spent several months in a psychiatric hospital, where he saw a very competent psychiatrist—the first doctor to take him seriously. He was diagnosed as having obsessive-compulsive disorder and given appropriate medication. This was in 1988. He got better, but was still not healthy.

On February 15, 1990, the FDA approved a new medication, Anafranil (clomipramine), and Bob was soon put on it. It controlled his disorder much more effectively. He is now on two medications, and is a successful practicing accountant.

Susie is philosophical about their experience. "It is the times and our culture. It causes even doctors to shy away from the real problem. And we were fortunate, because we were able to pay the enormous bills with the help of our parents. What about all those other people out there who don't have the money or the insurance to do what we had to do?"

Unfortunately, every day there are far too many people like Susie and Bob who have to deal with the onset of a mental illness in the family. Maybe you are one of them. How can you recognize the illness? What can you do? Where do you go for help?

There are so many questions to be answered. It may be reassuring to know that there are recognizable symptoms for the major mental illnesses. Once an illness can be identified, help is available.

Warning Signs of Mental Illness

I described the symptoms of each of the major illnesses in chapter 2. Of course, any of us could be affected by them at different times in our lives. How do you know when you're dealing with mental illness rather than a strong and normal reaction to a life crisis, a physical illness, a side effect of medication, or some other factor? The answer is, you don't. That's why an evaluation by a medical professional is necessary. If someone you love has persistent or extreme symptoms, follow your instincts and do what you can to persuade him or her to go for an evaluation.

It may be helpful for you to review the symptoms in chapter 2. Also, you can watch for these common warning signs[1]:

- Marked personality change over time
- Confused thinking; strange or grandiose ideas
- Prolonged severe depression; apathy; or extreme highs and lows
- Substance abuse

- Withdrawal from society
- Thinking or talking about suicide
- Anger or hostility out of proportion to the situation
- Delusions, hallucinations, hearing voices

Special Warning Signs in Younger Children

It can be more difficult to recognize mental health problems in children than in adults. But according to the American Academy of Child and Adolescent Psychiatry, these are some of the danger signals that indicate a child may need a professional evaluation for mental problems:

- Marked fall in school performance
- Poor grades in school despite trying very hard
- Extreme worry or anxiety, as shown by regular refusal to go to school, to sleep, or to take part in activities that are normal for the child's age
- Hyperactivity: fidgeting, constant movement beyond regular playing
- Persistent nightmares
- Persistent disobedience or aggression (longer than six months) and provocative opposition to authority figures
- Frequent, unexplainable temper tantrums

Special Warning Signs in Preadolescents and Adolescents

- Marked change in school performance
- Abuse of alcohol and/or drugs
- Inability to cope with problems and daily activities

- Marked changes in sleeping and/or eating habits
- Many complaints of physical ailments
- Consistent violation of rights of others; opposition to authority; truancy, thefts, vandalism
- Intense fear of becoming obese with no relationship to actual body weight
- Depression, shown by sustained, prolonged negative mood and attitude, often accompanied by poor appetite, difficulty sleeping, or thoughts of death
- Frequent outbursts of anger

So much of the time, symptoms for different illnesses overlap. For example, anxiety, depression, familial stress and abuse, and even middle-ear infections can all have symptoms that mimic those of ADHD (attention deficit hyperactivity disorder). And if undiagnosed or untreated, ADHD can trigger childhood depression, anxiety disorder, conduct disorder, and learning disabilities. So, if you suspect that your child or teenager has a mental health problem, be sure to get a careful diagnosis.

Warning Signs of Suicide

Since most suicides have been linked to mental illness, you must be especially vigilant if your loved one shows any of the following warning signs:

- Loses interest in activities and hobbies that were previously sources of pleasure
- Gives away favorite possessions, such as stamp collections, jewelry, or money
- Writes a will

- Has conversations that seem rational but have an unusually dark quality to them in which death is ennobled or elevated
- Makes oblique references to others who have died; although the death may have been tragic, there is a sense of identification or commiseration with the victim
- Writes poetry or prose laced with darkness, images of death, and profound loneliness
- Continuously and persistently discounts the positive and embraces the negative
- Increases alcohol or drug abuse
- Makes preparations and/or talks about a suicide plan that is concrete, specific, within means, and lethal—and there are no deterrents to prevent carrying out the plan. *This is a sign of great danger.* It is a myth that people who talk about suicide don't actually follow through!
- Seems detached from emotions and withdraws from friends or family
- Experiences a lifting of the depression. Ironically, those who are pulling out of depression can be at greater risk for suicide than those in deep depression. The lethargy inherent in depression may have dissipated but left behind suicidal thoughts. At this stage, a depressed individual has more energy to carry out a lethal plan.

You should also know that asking questions about suicide does not put ideas into someone's head—it does not cause the person to commit suicide. So if you or your family member is depressed, it is important to ask the following questions without worry about planting the idea:

- Have you been thinking a lot about death?
- Have you been wishing that you were dead or that you wouldn't wake up in the morning?

- Have you had thoughts about hurting yourself or killing someone?
- Have you made a plan to hurt yourself?[2]

If the answer to any of these questions is yes, you need to get help immediately.

If you recognize any of the above warning signs in someone you care about, or even yourself, remember that mental illness is a medical illness, and help is available. You may have to steer the ill one toward professional evaluation as Susie eventually did with Bob. And, if the troubled person is withdrawn or agitated, you may need to volunteer information about the condition to the professional making the assessment. *The most important thing you can do for a loved one is get professional help.*

Working Through Denial

Even though you may recognize that there is a problem, your loved one may be unwilling to admit it. Some who suffer are so affected by the symptoms that they are unable to ask for help. Others resist out of fear of being labeled "crazy" or feelings of shame. Given the stigma that has been associated with these illnesses for so many years, this reluctance is easy to understand, but it does not have to govern your actions.

You too, however, may be in denial. It is a common initial reaction to the shock of learning that a family member has a mental illness. But there is no reason to be ashamed—no one chooses to be mentally ill, and the disturbing behavior is not an act of will. As you will see in subsequent chapters, these illnesses are biological disorders that happen to affect the mind rather than the body.[3] *If someone you love is mentally ill or you suspect he or she is, don't pretend there is nothing wrong.* Offer your compassion and understanding, and get professional help!

Sometimes mentally ill individuals who desperately need help will refuse to go for treatment. If this happens with your loved one, you should look for a support group. Many others have had similar experiences, and they can offer valuable advice about ways to respond. You may also make an appointment for yourself, maybe at a community mental health center or with a private doctor, and ask for advice. Learn all about what is available in the community—about the mental health system, providers, programs, medications—so that you can be clear and, hopefully, persuasive in helping your family member accept the need for professional assistance. Even if your loved one completely refuses treatment, you must continue to seek support for yourself from those who understand and share your dilemma. Continue also to encourage and acknowledge any small steps the family member might make toward accepting treatment.

Finding the Right Help

Susie and Bob went through many harrowing experiences before they found the right therapist for Bob. This is a common occurrence. You may not know where to turn to find help either. These sources can be helpful in getting a recommendation:

- Your family doctor or clergy
- Friends and other family members
- Local psychiatric and psychological societies
- Local or state affiliates of national organizations such as NAMI or the NMHA (check the yellow pages to find these

organizations and other societies, agencies, etc. Also, see appendix D)

- Senior citizen centers or family service/social service agencies
- Your insurance company or HMO, which may have a list of participating therapists from which to choose
- Private or state hospitals with outpatient clinics
- A nearby university or teaching hospital that has a counseling center, or a psychiatry or psychology professor specializing in your loved one's illness (if you already have a diagnosis)
- The employee assistance counselor where you work
- Community mental health centers, where services are often available at low cost or on a sliding fee scale for those who are unable to pay high fees
- If the ill one is a child, the principal or school psychologist can be a good resource

Many people first consult their family doctor, and it is important to rule out any physical illness that could be causing the symptoms you or your loved one are experiencing. But family doctors are often not trained to recognize mental problems. And if you stay with the doctor, treatment will probably be medically based and short-term. I would urge you to see a mental health professional—and there are a wide variety to choose from. If you have not had to deal with the mental health system before, you may be confused about the options. The differences depend on the person's degree of education and training.

- *Psychiatrists.* Psychiatrists are physicians (M.D.s) who have graduated from medical school and have completed four additional years of training in psychiatry. In general, they are the only mental health professionals permitted to prescribe medication. Some psychiatrists focus on medications and deal exclusively with individuals with severe and persistent mental illnesses, while others conduct psychotherapy as well as prescribe medication.

• *Psychologists.* Psychologists have completed master's degrees and doctorates in psychology or counseling. Their degrees may read Ph.D., Psy.D., or Ed.D. Working with individuals, families, and children, they may be trained in many forms of therapy and must undergo two years of supervised internship after the completion of their doctorate.

• *Clinical Social Workers.* Social workers hold master's degrees (and sometimes Ph.D.s). Their training includes fieldwork in a wide range of human services, including mental health settings. They often focus upon the social context of their patients' lives. In most states, licensed clinical social workers (L.C.S.W. or C.S.W.) are required to undergo supervised training before they can conduct therapy with individuals and families.

• *Psychiatric Nurses.* Psychiatric nurses are registered nurses with additional training in psychiatry. They often work in mental health settings as part of a therapeutic team. Advanced practice nurses have a master's degree and can provide psychotherapy, and in some states may prescribe medication.

• *Marriage and Family Therapists.* These professionals usually hold master's degrees and have undergone supervised training. If you are considering seeing a marriage or family therapist, be sure that he or she is licensed. In many states anyone can say they offer marriage therapy or marriage counseling, even if they have not had appropriate training.

• *Clergy.* Pastoral counselors can offer psychological counseling within a religious context. They are not required to be licensed, but they may have received additional psychological training and may be certified by the American Association of Pastoral Counselors.[4]

How do you know which of these professionals is best for you? As you can see from the list above, only psychiatrists are medical doctors and are generally the only ones who can prescribe drugs. They can also recognize physical illnesses that might be causing your loved ones problems. Psychologists, social workers, and some psychiatric nurses offer lower-cost services, and in today's world of managed care, they are being favored more and more. All are trained to recognize mental illnesses, and all but some of the psychiatric nurses can provide therapy. They can all be most helpful in pointing you in the direction of the proper therapist. In fact, other professionals at mental health clinics, university hospitals, and such can steer you in the right direction. Since mental health professionals have different specialties, it is important that the therapist you choose specializes in the problem your loved one has.

The most critical element in choosing a therapist is the relationship that develops between the professional and the patient (and you, for that matter). All of us can almost instinctively tell when another person is interested in us, sensitive to the way we feel, compassionate, and truly cares about what happens to us. This is the kind of relationship that one must have with a therapist. After all, the patient will be sharing his or her most intimate thoughts and feelings with this professional, and if there is not a "good fit," very little progress will be made in treating the illness.

It is sometimes wise to shop for a therapist—to interview several before choosing one. It is important to get information about the therapist's credentials, specialties in treatment, and payment requirements. During the initial meeting between the patient and therapist, with or without you and other family members, the discussion may focus on what is happening in the life of the affected one, including the symptoms being experienced. Your loved one will be able to get a sense of whether or not there is a good patient/therapist connection. If the "fit" is not right, keep looking until the right one is found.

As the search begins, there are several things you need to keep in mind:

• Anyone can be called a "psychotherapist." This is not a legal term. Be sure to choose a mental health professional who is licensed by your state. This assures you that the individual has had extensive training, has participated in supervised practice, passed a rigorous state or national qualifying exam, and pursues continuing education.

• Ask if the individual is a member of the American Psychiatric Association, the American Psychological Association, or another nationally recognized group. These organizations have high membership standards.

• People often confuse the term psychiatrist, psychologist, and psychoanalyst. Psychoanalysts have been trained in a specialized program during which they have undergone psychoanalysis themselves. Psychoanalysis is a form of long-term psychotherapy originally developed and practiced by Sigmund Freud, but it is not the only form of psychotherapy available. Psychiatrists, psychologists, and clinical social workers can all receive psychoanalytic training, as can lay individuals who are not otherwise licensed.

• Many who are ill see more than one therapist at a time. They may be in counseling with a psychologist or social worker, for instance, while also seeing a psychiatrist for medication and periodic follow-up and blood tests to monitor their medication.

• If a professional brushes off your family member's complaints, as happened with Susie and Bob, seek out another. Don't give up if you know something is wrong.

• If a good relationship does not develop with the chosen therapist, feel free to try others. A "good fit," based on trust, is necessary for the best possible treatment and outcome.

Building a Partnership

It is important to recognize your role as a member of a team that will be helping your loved one and for you to build a partnership with the professionals involved. There are many ways in which you can assist, even with disorders as severe and debilitating as schizophrenia.

In *The Good News About Depression,* University of Florida psychiatrist Mark S. Gold explains, "The days of dealing directly with a patient, administering medication and/or therapy along with an occasional therapy session with the family, are gone. . . . The patient, the doctor, and the family are all part of the treatment plan, and that plan can't work if everyone involved doesn't understand what the treatment is and what to expect."[5] Your involvement is crucial.

The treatment team may include more than one professional, as I mentioned earlier, and sometimes there are staff members from a hospital, a residential program, or day care center that will be part of the team.

It may be that your ill family member has been hospitalized and discharged into your care. (It is not uncommon for a first encounter with mental health workers to be in the emergency room of a local hospital.) You will need to know what to expect and how to reduce the chance of future episodes. As part of the treatment team, you will be given information about outpatient services, medication schedules, future appointments, and so on. In some cases, families are not equipped to meet the varied and urgent needs of the discharged patient, so the team may help find a halfway house or a residential center.

Your role as a member of the team may be further defined during family therapy sessions. This kind of therapy involves the person who is ill and you—spouse, parents, siblings, and/or children—working together with one or more professionals. During the sessions each of you will have the opportunity to raise concerns and discuss how to better communicate with one another and deal with crises that may arise. You may also learn how to participate in the treatment plan and the patient's "homework" assignments, and you can receive needed support for yourself if you are feeling stressed by the illness.

Mental illness is a family affair, causing suffering among all family members. Dr. Richard A. Perlmutter of Johns Hopkins University explains that "addressing the pain, uncertainty, misconceptions, and fears of family members and involving them in treatment can be enormously helpful to the patient, to the family member, and to the process of recovery."[6]

When individuals are suffering from one of the major mental illnesses (schizophrenia, manic-depression, major depression), family therapy sessions that include the patient may or may not work. I met recently, for example, with the mother of a young man who has manic-depressive disorder. She told me that what she needed most, instead of family therapy, was "supportive family counseling"—education and practical, concrete advice from the team caring for her son. She sought information about the illness—the treatment, medication, and what to realistically expect about recovery; services available in the community; what to do in case of an emergency; details on legal procedures involved; and sources of financial assistance.

The team can also guide you to the many other families in your community who know and understand your plight based upon their own experiences. Support groups can be of enormous value (see chapter 11). Some hospitals offer these, as do local chapters of the National Alliance for the Mentally Ill, which exist in nearly every major city in the country. Remember that you are not alone. The more effort you put into building a strong support team for your family member, the more support you will find for yourself.

Treatment Options

Before your loved one begins treatment, you must be aware that there are no easy solutions to mental health problems. The treatment process may take a long time. Even the evaluation phase can take several sessions. The therapist will ask many questions: about family history, about the patient's earlier behavior, whether other relatives have had a mental disorder, if the patient is or has been employed, if he or she has good social relationships. There will also be questions for the family members about when they first noticed peculiar behavior and if some traumatic event had preceded it, such as a death or a divorce, the loss of a job, or a move away from familiar surroundings and friends. Although some of the questions may seem irrelevant, the therapist has a reason for asking them. Diagnosing mental illnesses is not easy. The symptoms of some are so similar that doctors sometimes find it hard to tell them apart. The more information they have, the better able they will be to determine the problem. The therapists may also administer personality or intelligence tests and will need the medical records of the person being evaluated.

Once a diagnosis is ventured, the treatment may include one or more of the following: psychotherapy, medication, or behavior therapy. Sometimes one will be effective, at other times a combination will be needed, depending on the symptoms and the diagnosis. To help you understand what to expect, I will briefly describe these options.

Psychotherapy

Often referred to as "talk therapy," psychotherapy is based on the premise that the patient's symptoms are the result of internal conflicts that can be relieved through in-depth discussions with the therapist. Sometimes the "talks" will focus on feelings and reactions to the problems of living, such as conflicts with other people and ways to improve relationships with those at home or on the job. At other times the talks will focus on conflicts from childhood that have long been repressed. "Homework" is often an important part of this type of therapy. It can help individuals remain active in therapy while encouraging them to apply what they have learned in the sessions to their "outside" lives. It also helps them feel more self-reliant.

Homework may consist of keeping a daily list of situations and the automatic thoughts they provoke, identifying and rating pleasurable experiences (to prove that life is worth living), reading material that pertains to the problems, writing, reviewing therapy sessions on tape, or role-playing.

Behavior Therapy

While psychotherapy focuses on changing thoughts, behavior therapy focuses on replacing negative "habits" with positive behavior. These therapies are action oriented. Remember Jerilyn Ross from chapter 2? She suffered from a panic disorder and was afraid to go above the tenth floor of a building. Working with her behavior therapist, going up one floor at a time—eventually to the top of a forty-four-story building—she was able to over-come the disorder.

Homework also plays an important role in behavior therapy. Depending on the diagnosis, the patient may be encouraged to return to doing things that were once pleasurable and to become more active socially. This may not be easy at first, but over a period of time, it can be very helpful in easing one back into normal social life.

Medications

As we have learned, medications have been greatly improved in recent years. They are effective for many types of mental illnesses and are the major treatment for the most severe ones. You will find more information about these in the chapters on the specific illnesses. The most important thing for you to know about medications is that once prescribed, they must be taken until the doctor says to stop, even if a patient begins to feel better. Some medications must be stopped gradually to give the body time to adjust; abrupt discontinuation can be very hazardous. And in some cases, such as schizophrenia, manic-depressive illness, and major depression, a loved one may need to take medications for the rest of his or her life to avoid recurrence of the disabling symptoms.

More Stories of Hope

Almost all mental illnesses can be improved with treatment. I am always hearing stories about people overcoming these illnesses:

• "I began behavior modification therapy and it turned my life around. It enabled me to be self-supporting and live a normal life, for which I am grateful."

• "After intensive therapies of various kinds—talk, art, dance—and a regimen of lithium, I was well and strong enough to begin taking the steps to achieve the fairly stable and happy life I now have."

• "In 1979, one twin daughter, twenty-eight years old, became ill with bipolar disorder; ten years later, our son (thirty-two years old, married, and the father of a two-year-old son) was hospitalized with the same disorder. So for almost twenty years, our family has experienced and survived all the dreadful consequences of brain disorders. . . .

"Between the two of them there have been a dozen hospitalizations. Each was divorced; our son lost custody of his son, and they have lost almost all of their old friends. Our son has been in two jails and we have paid out enormous legal fees. . . .

"Fortunately for our family, our story ends well. The rollercoaster ride produced by all the old medications that they tried has slowed. While not completely out of the woods, our daughter and son are now taking a new 'atypical psychotropic' medication and they have been stable since beginning it over three years ago. Some of the terrible side effects of older medications (hand tremors, sluggishness, loss of memory) have diminished or abated, so that our daughter now holds a part-time job in the office of a mental health advocacy organization, and our son is trying to return to college."

• "Learning to manage my mental illness through self-help and the use of the latest medications has given me a quality of life I didn't think was possible just a few years ago."

• "The trauma lived inside me and finally overcame me and I really hardly knew where I was or what I was doing all those years. I was hallucinating off the walls and I thought I was going crazy. It was all so horrible . . . some call me the Prozac Kid, because that's what did it for me, with the help of my wife and family . . . now I'm back at work. I haven't missed a day in four years. . . .

"God has given me back my life, and because of God I can come home in the afternoon and look up on my deck and there stands a beautiful little twelve-year-old girl with a basketball in her hand. She smiles, looks at me and says, 'Kid, do you want to play a little one-on-one?' "

Accepting the Role of Medication

According to the guidelines of the American Psychiatric Association, patients with mild to moderate depression can benefit from psychotherapy alone. The therapy should decrease the symptoms of the illness, reduce the risk of relapse, and improve the patient's quality of life. However, should symptoms persist for more than twenty sessions or should they worsen during that time, then medication is recommended and is often necessary for recovery.

Pulitzer Prize–winning newspaper columnist Art Buchwald, who himself has suffered from depression, addressed this issue in a 1996 radio broadcast with his friends Mike Wallace and William Styron.[7]

"If you'd say to someone who has a bad back, 'Take this pill,' they'll take it immediately," Buchwald explained. "But people who have depression want to fight it without any help because they think that's the way to lick it. And all the people that I know that have been in serious trouble are those who refused to take Prozac, Zoloft . . . because they feel they've given in. And I think that's a very important message to people. The pills are there, there's a reason for them. There's enough proof that they work for a lot of people."

"The pills are there . . . they work for a lot of people." Yet many are confused by myths about medications. Some believe that pills are a "crutch," that they will become dependent on them, that they rob them of their personalities, that they are addictive, or are tranquilizers. None of these statements is true for most of the modern medications, even including those for schizophrenia.

Some people with mental illness may have to take medication for the rest of their lives, but so do those who have diabetes or high blood pressure. I have a thyroid problem, and I have to take a Synthroid pill every day. I don't consider it a crutch. Would anyone consider insulin or high blood pressure medication a crutch? Would we fear becoming addicted to these medications? Of course not. They help improve our quality of life.

Once individuals begin on a course of medication, it may take several weeks to reach its full effect. This is especially true for those used to treat depression and anxiety disorders. If one of them produces unwanted side effects, there are very often alternatives that can work just as well without the side effects. Sometimes it can take several months to find the right "fit" between the individual and the treatment. Your loved one may have to try different medications in varying doses before finding which works best. Setbacks can be frustrating and time-consuming, and the ongoing monitoring can take longer than you want, but with realistic expectations, you will be able to weather the process well.

Dual Diagnosis

Many families know how difficult it is to find treatment for their mentally ill relatives who also abuse drugs or alcohol. If your loved one has both problems, you will find that programs that treat people with mental illnesses usually do not treat substance abusers, and programs for substance abusers are not geared for people with mental illness. Affected individuals often bounce from one place to another, or are refused treatment by single-diagnosis programs.

The presence of both disorders must first be established by careful assessment by a medical doctor and mental health professional. This may be difficult because the symptoms of one problem can mimic the symptoms of the other. Once the assessment confirms the dual diagnosis, you should work with mental health professionals on a strategy to integrate care and find incentives for getting the ill one into treatment.

If your loved one is addicted to drugs and/or alcohol, experts offer the following advice:

• Don't regard it as a family disgrace. Recovery from an addiction is possible just as with other illnesses.

• Don't nag, preach, or lecture to an addict/alcoholic. Chances are he or she has already heard or knows everything you can say. You may only increase his or her need to lie or make promises that cannot be kept.

• Guard against having a "holier than thou" or martyrlike attitude.

• Don't use the "if you loved me" approach. It is like saying "If you loved me, you would not have tuberculosis."

• Avoid threats unless you think them through carefully and definitely intend to carry them out. Idle threats only make the alcoholic/addict feel you don't mean what you say.

• Don't hide the alcohol/drugs or dispose of them. Usually this only pushes the addict into a state of desperation.

• Don't let the addict/alcoholic persuade you to drink or use drugs. Condoning the drinking/using lets the ill one put off seeking help.

• Don't be jealous of the method of recovery the alcoholic/addict chooses. You may feel left out when he or she turns to other people for help in staying sober. If someone needed medical care, you wouldn't be jealous of the doctor.

• Don't expect an immediate, 100 percent recovery. In any illness, there is a period of convalescence. There may be relapses and times of tension and resentment.

• Don't try to protect the recovering person from drinking/using. The person must learn to say no gracefully.

• Don't do for the alcoholic/addict that which he or she can do. Don't remove the problem before he or she can face it, solve it, or suffer the consequences.

• Do offer love, support, and understanding in the recovery.[8]

Dealing with Noncompliance

Noncompliance means not following doctor's orders. As a member of the treatment team, you have an important role in encouraging your loved one to continue going to therapy and taking medication that has been prescribed. Sometimes the side effects of drugs make people want to stop, but there are other reasons, too.

Patients with schizophrenia may decide to avoid follow-up treatment and stop taking their medication, believing the voices that tell them treatment is not necessary. This can lead to the return of more severe psychotic symptoms. People who are depressed, like Rod Steiger, may discontinue their medication when they begin feeling better, only to fall back into a depression when their brain chemistry becomes unbalanced once more. Or, in their pessimistic state, they may believe that nothing—not even medication—will help them.

In *An Unquiet Mind,* professor of psychiatry and herself a sufferer of bipolar illness, Kay Redfield Jamison writes about her resistance to taking lithium for manic-depressive illness. It wasn't so much the side effects—the loss of coordination, the difficulty reading, the memory lapses—as it was the longing for the highs of her manic periods that had seemed to give her life so much color. Now, with the highs gone, her life had become dull.

Jamison notes that it's hard for those with manic-depressive illness to relinquish "the positive aspects of the illness that can arise during the milder manic states: heightened energy and perceptual awareness, increased fluidity and originality of thinking, intense exhilaration of moods and experience, increased sexual desire, expansiveness of vision, and a lengthened grasp of aspiration. . . . These intoxicating experiences were highly addictive in nature and difficult to give up."

Here is where your partnership with the doctor is critical. According to Dr. Mark S. Gold, 20 to 25 percent of all hospital admissions for depression result from noncompliance. "Family members can help immeasurably," he writes, "by encouraging compliance with the doctor's orders and by keeping track."[9] Your encouragement may help a loved one avoid the common cycle that so many who are mentally ill experience—going off medication, spiraling out of control, needing emergency treatment, and being remedicated. In chapter 6, you will read about Sam, a young man with schizophrenia, whose mother and sister worked closely with him and his physician to make sure he took his medicine after he was released from the hospital. Although not every story has such a happy ending, the family's involvement made the critical difference in Sam's recovery, and you can play that role, too.

Chapter 5

After the Diagnosis: Managing Workplace, Financial, Legal, and Other Matters

Mental Illness and the Workplace

Once those with mental illness have sought professional help and have their illness under control, they may be ready to look for work. Some may be looking for a job for the first time; others may have had their employment interrupted by the illness.

Recently, newspaper columnist Ann Landers printed the letter of a man who had been diagnosed with and successfully treated for manic-depression. Formerly the vice president of a large company, M.K. was dismissed from his job when his illness led him to yell at the chairman of the board. Although treatment with lithium had helped him recover, when he called his old boss about returning to work he received no sympathy, either from the boss or from his coworkers.[1]

Like all of us, people with mental illnesses benefit from working, and they should not be denied that option if they are capable of carrying out their duties. Work fulfills many needs. It creates structure and meaning in our lives, gives us a sense of accomplishment, provides income and security, and also affords us the chance to socialize with friends and colleagues and to feel as if we belong to a community.

Your family member, like M.K., may encounter difficulties on the job, as do many others. According to an April 1997 report, more than 13 percent of complaints filed with the Equal Employment Opportunity Commission (EEOC) alleged discrimination resulting from emotional or psychiatric impairments.[2] The Americans with Disabilities Act of 1990 (ADA) mandates that businesses with fifteen employees or more cannot discriminate against a qualified job candidate or employee on the basis of a disability and must make reasonable accommodations for employees who suffer from mental disorders. These can include:

- Allowing for extra time off (for medical appointments)
- Altering work schedules (to accommodate someone on antidepressants, for example, who may be groggy in the morning). However, people with manic-depressive illness are well advised *not* to do changing shift work because it can interfere with their sleep/wake cycles. Sleep deprivation may trigger mania
- Making physical changes in the workplace, such as adding partitions or soundproofing for someone who has difficulty concentrating, or putting a desk by the window for a person who grows depressed if there is too little light

Guidelines issued by the EEOC also require an employer to provide a temporary job coach to help in the training of a qualified individual with a mental disability. And employers may not exclude a person who is mentally ill from job eligibility unless they can prove that the exclusion is job related and "consistent with business necessity." They are not, however, required to excuse the behavior of an employee who threatens a coworker, even if the behavior results from a disorder. The ADA provides that anyone who feels discriminated against in the workplace because of mental illness can contact the EEOC at 800-669-4000 for assistance.

Many who are afflicted are reluctant to reveal a mental illness to a supervisor or employee assistance program where they work for fear of being stigmatized. Some progressive companies, such as Southwest Airlines and First Chicago Corporation, have been trying to solve this problem. They have trained their managers to spot the signs of depression, gently broach the subject with employees, and suggest possible resources within the company. Others, like General Telephone & Electronics and Delta Airlines, have changed their health insurance plans to provide for early treatment of mental illness. Many companies offer confidential 800-number hotlines for workers who don't know where to turn with their emotional problems.[3]

Those who became mentally ill as adolescents and are just now entering the workforce may not know where to turn for help. For them, a "supported employment" agency that has a proven track record and is sensitive to mental health consumer issues is a valuable resource. Supported employment is what we would call "real work in a real workplace" for those with the most severe disabilities. Individuals work for pay in businesses alongside nonhandicapped people. Job coaches, usually from a mental health center, go with them to work, help them learn the ropes, stay with them until they no longer need the support.

One of the best programs I know is the Green Door in Washington, D.C. Begun as a small secondhand clothes business to provide work for severely mentally ill people (called members), it has grown into a model program that now offers residential facilities and a clubhouse.

Members begin their job training by gaining skills at the clubhouse. They learn to use the office equipment and food service appliances there. Next, they get on-the-job experience in part-time, paid jobs with transitional employers (partners of the program who agree to hire the members). The members are trained for these positions by Green Door staff and paid by the employer. The employer is guaranteed a job well done each day. If for some reason a member can't work on a given day, Green Door staff will substitute. After several transitional jobs, members have the training they need and are then helped to get permanent jobs, where they are still supported by the Green Door staff as needed.

Renee McPherson, a member, wrote an article she called "Working My Way Up" for the fall 1997 issue of *Green Door News:*

> At Green Door I worked in the Café Unit where I learned to use the cash register and purchase food wholesale. I learned how to use the computer and the copier. After a while, I began to feel more confident.
>
> Green Door put me on temporary group jobs with other members. After that, I worked two transitional jobs at the Public Welfare Foundation and the American Psychological Association. These jobs helped prepare me for a permanent job. Now, I have a permanent job at Ottenberg Bakery as a Customer Service Representative, where I do data entry, take phone orders and handle customers' concerns.
>
> I like the way Green Door is set up. If you want to do something for yourself, there is opportunity and the door is open for you. It has helped to prepare me for society.

And Gina Lutz of Ottenberg Bakery says, "I can't say enough good things about Green Door. Their employment program instills a sense of self-worth and esteem in our employees. Green Door member Kim Foley [who gets thirty calls an hour from customers placing orders, fielding complaints, etc.] holds the highest call average without error in our division. Ottenberg is thrilled to be a part of the program."

Friends may be able to recommend helpful programs, and consumer advocacy organizations such as the National Mental Health Association and the National Alliance for the Mentally Ill also offer guidance and referrals to community employment agencies.

For those like M.K., who once held a responsible position and need help in finding new employment, I have included a list of employment resources in appendix D. Some individuals may require retraining. Others simply need help finding their way once more. When a job is found, the new worker must be encouraged to:

- Continue with therapy and keep his or her life in balance
- Focus on the positive aspects of work: financial security, independence, personal satisfaction
- Recognize the influence of office politics and personalities
- View barriers merely as inconveniences and setbacks as challenges to be overcome
- Develop a personal vision and strategy for his or her career
- Understand the illness and its symptoms and develop ways to minimize its effects on job performance
- Find out more about the Americans with Disabilities Act and the rights of mentally ill employees[4]

Insurance and Managed Care

There are many questions that need to be answered—for all of us, and particularly for you with your mentally ill family member—about the directions managed care is taking. Among them: How does one strike a balance among cost, quality care, and access to care? Will access to care be improved? Will quality of care be preserved? Will treatment results be based on the outcomes—whether or not the patient is helped—rather than on what insurance happens to cover or on cost containment. We in the mental health field are particularly concerned about these issues because of the historic discrimination in insurance coverage and the low quality of much institutional care for those who suffer from mental illnesses.

At one of our annual symposia at The Carter Center we talked about these issues. Among all of those present—consumers of mental health services, family members, providers, payers, managed care executives, and state Medicaid and mental health officials—there was general agreement with one of our speakers, nationally recognized economist Karen Davis,[5] who said, "Managed care offers the potential of improved access and quality through new emphasis on primary care, prevention, integration, and coordination of care for those with chronic or complex disease. . . . However, in today's market-driven environment, we have little ability to assure that care is managed in the interest of patients."

This is particularly important for mental health services. Senator Paul Wellstone (D-Minn.), who is concerned about the takeover of Medicaid by managed care, said in September of 1997, "Appropriate treatment for mental illness is not always a magic bullet where there's one procedure or one operation or one thing that can be done that will nurture people and enable people to be fully participating members of their community and to work with dignity." He added, "Sometimes you need more care. All too often people get denied that care."

Managed care has been applauded by those who pay for health care in the public and private sector alike for having slowed the health care cost spiral, but there is a growing sentiment that some managed care plans have cut costs at the expense of providing adequate coverage.[6]

Today, more than three quarters (77 percent) of all employees covered under an employer plan participate in some form of managed care. These plans have replaced traditional fee-for-service health insurance as the primary means of providing employer-sponsored health benefits in America. While virtually all plans provide some mental health and substance abuse coverage, the level and scope of coverage varies widely.

I made a speech in September 1997 to an annual meeting of employee benefit managers, stressing the importance of mental health coverage for employees in their companies. Not only does it make for a happier, healthier workplace, but it is cost-effective—resulting in less absenteeism, less turnover of jobs, greater productivity, and higher quality of work. In addition, companies that have provided these services have seen their overall health care cost come down after a few years. It has been found, for example, that when people have help with illnesses such as depression and anxiety disorders, they seek fewer general health services.

At W. C. Bradley Company in Columbus, Georgia, where about twelve hundred full-time employees make Char-Broil grills, mental health coverage has been a priority since 1975. "We were trying to encourage employees and dependents to seek counseling help, with the idea that mental and emotional health have a great impact on physical health," says chief executive officer Steve Butler. "We didn't want any barriers for employees."

While mental health costs rose, the company's overall health care costs per employee were as much as 30 percent *below* those of other area companies. "Primary care physicians have told us an awful lot of visits they see are actually mental health issues, rather than physical health," Rick Woodham, a company executive, said.[7]

A few years ago, Digital Equipment Corporation insisted that their managed mental health plans remove all predetermined restrictions on care. This means that their employees can receive therapy alone or therapy plus medication for as long as they need it. In effect, Digital replaced blanket across-the-board restrictions with the careful management of care on a case-by-case basis.

"The HMOs thought we were crazy at first," recalls Digital benefits manager Fran Bastien. "They thought costs would go sky-high." In fact, Digital reduced its total health care cost by $100 million over four years.

Federal Express also provides its employees with flexible comprehensive mental health and substance abuse benefits. So do other forward-looking national corporations like McDonnell Douglas, Chevron, Honeywell, Pacific Bell, and IBM.

As with any system, there are some really good programs and some that are not so good. One day I was in my office in Atlanta when I got a call from a young man who was suicidal. He had not been feeling well for some time but had continued trying to work and do a good job, even being selected employee of the year at one point. Finally, he had requested time off to see a doctor. He was referred to the company's HMO. After being shuffled from one doctor to another, he was sent to a psychiatrist who simply asked him, "What's wrong? What do you want to do about it? What kind of medication do you want?" That was it!

After the visit to the psychiatrist, the young man went home and went to bed. A friend found him there and suggested that he call me. After listening to his story of managed care at its worst, I got in touch immediately with officials at the HMO and was able to get some good help for him.

There are many complaints about the way managed care systems treat people with mental illnesses: that they don't provide the new antipsychotic medications as a first line of treatment;

that hospital stays are limited and even denied for patients who are noncompliant and disruptive—common features of severe mental illnesses; that they don't respond to suicide attempts with immediate care; that privacy and confidentiality of patients' medical records are jeopardized; that case managers, though not therapists themselves, overrule recommendations of patients' psychiatrists; that medical decisions are dictated by cost, not quality.[8]

One young woman expressed her concerns over privacy and confidentiality in a letter to the editors at *Newsweek*. She was told by a managed mental health care company that in order to receive coverage of her treatment for mental illness, she would have to allow detailed accounts of her therapy sessions to be seen by nonmedical personnel. She feared her medical records could be made available to people unqualified to evaluate them.

The correspondent never returned to the managed care provider; instead, she resumed therapy with her original psychiatrist, shouldering the full cost herself. If you and your loved one find yourselves in this kind of situation, you may have to fight with your insurance company for the consideration you need. Getting support from advocacy groups can be helpful. A good place to start is with the Mental Health Insurance Hot Line of the NMHA. You can call them at 800-933-9896. Or call NAMI at 800-950-NAMI (6264).

Managed care has taken over so quickly that there are bound to be missteps, but we're going to have to find ways to make it work, since so many of us are covered by this kind of insurance, and our numbers are growing every day. Managed care has grown so fast that regulations have not caught up with it. But there are some hopeful signs.

An article in *The New York Times* (July 14, 1997) illustrates how managed care may be forced to change in the near future. The report outlined California's plans for a wholesale review of its managed care system. The governor and legislators, under the weight of consumer complaints, provider activism, and pressure from various groups such as the elderly, have formed a joint commission to "recommend improvements in managed care." The article also described "an avalanche of proposals" going to the state senate and assembly that would regulate managed care more tightly.

One individual wrote, in the September 5, 1997, issue of *Psychiatric News,* that rather than claiming "we are winning" or "we are losing" the battle with managed care companies, "I believe 'we are changing' is closer to reality." He continued, "Addressing managed care issues, state legislators across the country have introduced about 1,000 managed-care-related bills just this year. At least 182 have already become law compared with only 100 in 1996. In June, the New Jersey legislature approved a bill that would establish an independent appeals process for HMO members who have had treatment denied." He goes on to describe one of the many bills before the California legislature: a consumer-sponsored, eleven-point patients' bill of rights.

Of major concern for those who suffer from severe and persistent mental illness is whether managed care can ever provide the full array of services that the government now provides. And are these services in jeopardy? Although funds are always short and government services are never as sufficient as we would like them to be, Medicaid programs for eligible mentally ill individuals now offer help with housing, rehabilitation services, finding employment, etc. Advocates have fought hard for these services over the years. There needs to be a careful look into efforts of managed care companies to contract with state governments to provide oversight of these services.

This, and the fact that too much emphasis has been put on cost containment at the expense of the quality of services, worries all of us. I hope that more attention will be paid to the outcomes of treatments; careful measurement and reporting of these outcomes will help create a proper balance between cost containment and the quality of services in managed care plans.

Advocacy groups have organized to have input into changes that need to be made, to become partners in the decision-making process. As Laurie Flynn of NAMI says, "We NAMI families know what good services look like, and we've fought hard to get them . . . managed care companies must not be allowed to deny us the future we deserve."

Let's not forget that there are some very good programs in the country. We're proud of the programs at Digital, McDonnell Douglas, W. C. Bradley, and the Bank of Chicago. Can all programs be as responsive?

Legal Issues

To be prepared for any kind of emergency, you should learn all you can about the legal issues that you may encounter with a mentally ill family member. You can check with your state authorities about the laws that govern these issues. Also, patients-rights advocates, public defenders, the Legal Aid Society, private attorneys, and others can provide advice.

Most current laws regarding involuntary hospitalization, informed consent, confidentiality, and the rights of people with mental illness reflect efforts to correct some of the abuses of the past. While we should be pleased with such progress, it must be acknowledged that, at times, people with mental illness and their families feel frustrated by the laws—but not always for the same reasons.

For example, current laws governing involuntary commitment to a hospital give more control to the consumer (the person with mental illness). While consumers believe these changes are necessary to protect their individual rights, family members may be frustrated when they try to get help for a severely mentally ill family member who doesn't want it. While laws vary from state to state, they are all based on the principle that individuals should be committed involuntarily only when they are a danger to themselves or others. Some family members feel this criterion is too strict and should be changed to include commitment upon serious relapse in persons with documented histories of severe and persistent mental illness.

Confidentiality is another area where there is often a difference of views between patients and their family members. In order to maintain trust and create a safe environment, a therapist will hold in confidence everything revealed in private sessions. The therapist is bound by law to do so and will break confidentiality only in special cases, such as threats of suicide or violence, or suspicion of child or elder abuse. Otherwise, without express written consent from the patient, the therapist cannot share information about treatment, not even with other mental health professionals.

This often poses a terrible dilemma for those caring for persons with psychotic disorders. When I asked one mother about the problem, she told me that families are not interested in the private conversations between the person and his or her therapist. But, she said, "What we need is basic information such as diagnosis, treatment plans, and medications in order to do a better job of caregiving—the same information that insurance companies are receiving."

She was visibly distressed about the issue, explaining further, "The Hippocratic oath has two ethical principles that apply here: One is that the physician [health care provider] protect the privacy of conversations so patients will trust them and continue to share information in the future; the other is that the physician must act in the best interest of the patient.

"There is a great deal of attention shown towards the first and very little towards the second. It is in the 'best interest of the patient' to share basic information with caregivers who often provide care twenty-four hours a day in their homes, without quiet rooms, extra medications, or staff shift changes. It is cruel and neglectful to shut out family caregivers from basic information."

We can all readily understand the genuine concern of such a family caregiver and also sense the ethical dilemma of the professional caregiver. Some states have passed laws that specify that limited information can be provided to family caregivers, but most have not yet done so. It appears that this issue will continue to be affected by the laws of each state, unless a federal law addresses it.

Finding the right balance between knowing enough to be helpful and protecting your family member's privacy is critical to effective treatment. You can ask the patient to sign a waiver, so that the therapist can share pertinent information with you. If the patient withholds permission, you can put your observations in writing. An "FYI" letter to the therapist might state, "You may not know she has stopped taking her medication," ". . . has been threatening to hurt herself," ". . . has been yelling at her coworkers."[9] It is always wise, though, to consult with the patient before sending the therapist any information, as some patients will resent communication without their okay.

If your loved one makes any suicidal statements or gestures, you must communicate this immediately to the therapist. Because of the confidentiality laws, the therapist may not be able to share the patient's response with you, but you will have done all you can to convey your concerns.

In the case of minors, these rules do not apply. As parents, you are the ultimate holders of confidentiality. However, if your teenager has revealed drug or early sexual activity to the therapist, the therapist may decide not to reveal this directly to you, but will ask instead for a family session during which the adolescent can be gently encouraged to bring up these issues.

What if your family member is too incapacitated to make reasonable decisions? In *Helping Yourself Help Others,* I explain that a person who is ill should sign a durable power of attorney allowing someone else—an "agent" or "attorney-in-fact," most likely you—to have permanent access to bank accounts and the power to make important property-related and financial decisions. You should see that such an agreement is signed by your loved one before it is actually needed so it can go into effect when a crisis occurs. How much or how little control to give to the "agent" can be spelled out, and the agreement can be canceled at any time. A durable power of attorney for health decisions can also be signed, specifying who should act on the patient's behalf in medical matters.

Guardianship or conservatorship is a more drastic measure in which the court declares an individual "incompetent" and appoints guardians or conservators to take charge of that person's interests. This is an all-or-nothing measure—either an individual is competent or not—and it can create harsh feelings among family members. You would be wise to consult an attorney if you wish to deal with your situation in this way.

Parents of severely mentally ill children often worry about who will care for their offspring after they are gone. Most people leave all of their assets to their spouse or children. But if the surviving individuals are mentally incompetent, the inheritance can be placed in a discretionary trust. Trustees can be instructed on how to care for the ill one upon your death. Again, an attorney can explain these options to you in greater detail.

Other Ways to Be Helpful

When someone you love has a mental illness, your involvement can be crucial in his or her treatment and recovery.

As mentioned, you can do "homework"—keeping a log of symptoms you are observing, the medications being taken, and the effectiveness of treatments and their side effects. By identifying the symptoms and results, you may be able to note early signs of relapse (such as increased withdrawal or changes in eating or sleeping patterns) and help your family member take steps to avert a full-blown episode of his or her mental disorder.

You can also be helpful in showing empathy and support. One day I was running an errand in town and ran into a friend who was suffering from depression. She told me she had been having a rough time and that none of her family thought she was really sick. She said, "They all say I could snap out of it if I wanted to. But it's not that easy. I wish they could understand that." What she needed was someone in the family to say "I know it's not easy for you right now" or "It must be terrible to feel that way." A kind word or caring gesture can have a very positive impact.

Dr. Mitch Golant, a Los Angeles–based clinical psychologist, explains in *What to Do When Someone You Love Is Depressed* that empathizing is important, but that you must also reassure the individual that he or she will not be abandoned. He suggests that family members say "I want you to know that you matter to me and you matter to the family. We'll get through this hopeless feeling together."[10] This will reassure a depressed person whose worst fear may be that of abandonment.

Another suggestion came from a mother who told me she had learned after many years that the best way to get along with her ill son was to be respectful, even when she was angry and wanted to lash out. She said that it had taken her a long time, but she had finally accepted the fact that he was mentally ill, and that his tormenting symptoms caused him to do things that neither he nor she understood. She tries to remember that at all times. It's not easy.

There are other ways you can be helpful. Encourage your family member to exercise and take walks. Videos of comedies can be helpful; music and religious services often lift the spirits. You might also encourage participation in activities formerly enjoyed, such as hobbies, sports, or cultural events. But be tender. Too much pressure can reinforce feelings of failure.

If your loved one suffers from psychosis (which can be a symptom of schizophrenia, manic-depressive illness, or severe depression), you may not know how to respond to the irrational statements or beliefs. The NIMH suggests that rather than going along with the delusions, you can say, "I don't see things the same way" or "I don't agree with your conclusions," while acknowledging that things may seem the way they do to the one who is ill.[11]

You can also praise any progress being made, even if at times it seems like only "baby steps" toward recovery. As the NIMH makes clear, "a positive approach may be helpful and perhaps more effective in the long run than criticism."

Keeping the mental illness a secret from other family members and friends can heighten everyone's feelings of shame, isolation, and stigma—even if the ill one insists that you not tell. And it can be exhausting for you. As a rule, honesty is always the best policy. Otherwise, it's easy to find yourself going along with the cover-up. Dr. Golant says that "most important, you and your loved one need to talk to each other about how best to convey the true nature of the [mental illness] without being destructive to your relationship."[12] After all, the illness affects the whole family; you're in it together. Once you do feel comfortable discussing it with others, be clear about the diagnosis and treatment, and ask for support: "Fred has been diagnosed with schizophrenia. We're working closely with the doctors to find the right medication. We hope we can count on your support," or, "Beverly is clinically depressed. It's not her fault, and it's not something she can 'snap out of.' We're trying different medications and are committed to helping her recover. We could use your help in keeping Beverly's attitude as positive as possible."

Rex Dickens has written some additional helpful reminders for the NAMI Sibling and Adult Children Network that I'd like to share with you:

- You cannot cure a mental disorder for a family member.
- The disorder may be periodic, with times of improvement and deterioration independent of your hopes or actions.
- It is as hard for the individual to accept the disorder as it is for other family members.
- A delusion will not go away by reasoning and therefore needs no discussion.
- Separate the person from the disorder. Love the person even if you hate the disorder.
- Acknowledge the remarkable courage your family member may show in dealing with a mental disorder.
- Strange behavior is a symptom of the disorder. Don't take it personally.
- Don't be afraid to ask your family member if he is thinking about suicide. . . . Discuss it to avoid it happening.
- It is natural to experience a cauldron of emotions such as grief, guilt, fear, anger, sadness, hurt, confusion, etc. You, not the ill member, are responsible for your own feelings.
- Eventually you may see the silver lining in the storm clouds: increased awareness, sensitivity, receptivity, compassion, maturity, and [becoming] less judgmental, self-centered.

Patience

Recovery from mental illness is often a two-steps-forward-one-step-back process. It requires patience from all concerned. Dylan Abraham, a consumer advocate for NAMI, explained this eloquently in a recent essay:

> Many times . . . and this is true for me . . . doctors, family, friends, and society in general try to rush the individual who is ill to come back in a hurry and "catch up" on the time they have "lost." This urging happens often, and it may be a tragic mistake to try to come back so fast. Recovery is important when someone is mentally ill, but it's not smart to turn recovery into a race with the clock. Getting well is not a race. It is something that takes time, patience, and a few ups and downs . . . people who are going through the trauma of such illnesses need to take small bites—not one huge bite—to be on their way again. With time, things will come around."[13]

Part II

New Treatments, New Hope

President George Bush declared the 1990s the "Decade of the Brain," and it is certainly living up to its promise. Within the past ten years, advances in our understanding of the brain have been amazing. The National Institute of Mental Health estimates that approximately 95 percent of what we know about the brain today has been learned only in the last decade.

This three-pound organ is the seat of the mind, the originator of normal and abnormal behaviors. There are about one hundred billion nerve cells in the brain and hundreds of trillions of connections among them. Across these connections, nerve cells communicate with one another, using more than one hundred different chemicals, including serotonin and dopamine. Every day scientists are making more and more progress in understanding this extraordinarily complex organ and the way it functions. In fact, there is a revolution going on in our understanding of mental illnesses, fueled by these new discoveries.

For many years, scientists waged a "nature versus nurture" debate about brain development. One side held that the brain was largely determined biologically at birth and could not be altered throughout one's lifetime, while the other believed that environment and parenting were of supreme importance and biology was of relatively little consequence. Today, most experts realize that nature *and* nurture are intertwined in brain development. They are not antagonists, but partners in building the brain.

We now know that the brain has an amazing capacity to change in response to its environment. Experiences and learning, medications, substance abuse, and probably prenatal "events" and infectious diseases may all play a role in altering brain circuits. Nerve cells may grow, shrink, or develop new connections, depending on what one learns or remembers. The activity of these cells can change the brain's structure, causing certain areas to enlarge while others diminish. This ability of the brain to change is called "plasticity." It means that nature and nurture interact in myriad ways to shape the perpetually developing brain.

Consider the case of depression. Continually having pessimistic thoughts after the death of a loved one can actually change the chemistry of the brain, which, in turn, can bring on a depressive episode in someone who is genetically vulnerable. As the NIMH explains, "People are not merely puppets pulled by the strings of biological processes; behavioral, mental, and social factors have powerful . . . effects on biological function."

Discoveries such as these and the ones I will outline next will lead to a clearer understanding of the origins of mental illnesses and better treatments for these disorders. And they will help free sufferers and their families from the oppression of stigma and the associated feelings of guilt that surround them.

Neurosciences: The New Sciences of the Brain

Imagine being able to peer into the living brain while it is actually functioning—without using a scalpel! Imagine being able to take photos of a normal brain and compare it to the brain of an individual with schizophrenia or obsessive-compulsive disorder. Imagine being able to pinpoint the precise location of an individual nerve cell among the billions that make up the brain.

All of this and more is happening today in the field of neuroscience, as researchers study how the nervous system works and how it is affected by disease. They are hoping to solve the age-old mystery of the brain's relationship to consciousness—to normal and abnormal human thought and behavior. And they are making great strides.

Because of the technological breakthroughs, for instance, scientists can study the individual components of nerve cells (*neurons*) that allow them to communicate; they can even detect which of our genes are active and which are "turned off" in a single cell. They can trace the connections of cells that create the "circuits" that underlie our mental lives, and with new imaging technologies, they can see these circuits at work in living human beings.

New imaging techniques have opened vast areas for exploration of the brain:

- CAT scans use computers to combine a series of X-rays to provide a clearer picture of the brain's structure than just the X-rays alone. But these are still static pictures.

- PET and SPECT scans reveal brain activity while it is occurring by measuring the amount of blood flow or the way glucose (blood sugar) is used in a region in the brain. The amount of blood flowing or glucose is directly related to the activity in that area. Thus PET and SPECT give us dynamic pictures of the brain at work.
- MRI scans are the newest way of studying the brain at work. Unlike PET or SPECT, which require radioactivity, MRI uses magnetic fields to probe brain activity. This technology is giving us almost miraculously clear pictures of the brain at work. Older, static MRI can give us clear information about any abnormalities in the structure of the brain.

These new tools give us dramatic views of the actual workings of the brain, and can reveal abnormalities associated with certain mental illnesses. Scientists, for example, have found subnormal activity in certain areas of the brain in people who are depressed and "hot spots" of abnormally high activity in the brains of those with obsessive-compulsive disorder.

Scans can also show which parts of the brain are activated when people with schizophrenia have visual and auditory hallucinations. These hallucinations are quite real to the sufferers and are produced in the very same areas of the brain in which we normally perceive sight and sound. The benefits of treatment can also be seen with these techniques; the scans show the brain function normalizing with appropriate medication and psychotherapy. The miracle of these neuroimaging scans is that they are noninvasive.

In the past we could only guess how the brain functioned, but today we can actually see which regions are involved in learning, memory, and behavior. Particular areas "light up" on the scans during these activities. As Steven Hyman, the director of the NIMH, has explained, "For the first time, we can see the thinking, feeling, living human brain."

There have also been breakthroughs in our understanding of the brain's chemistry. With the help of MRI scans, researchers now know that nerve cells communicate by constantly bombarding one another with chemicals. These chemicals, called *neurotransmitters,* attach themselves to adjacent cells much like a key fitting into a lock in order to send their messages. They have even been called "chemical messengers."[1]

Each neurotransmitter has specific *receptors* to which it will attach on an adjoining cell, and each cell can have many different receptors for different neurotransmitters. Some neurotransmitters excite nerve cells to action, while others dampen their activity. Yet others produce complex changes in the chemistry of the receiving cell.

Disturbances in the levels of certain neurotransmitters have been associated with specific mental illnesses. In schizophrenia there is good evidence that the neurotransmitter dopamine, and perhaps serotonin as well, are not working right.[2] (We will become familiar with these two neurotransmitters because they play a role, especially serotonin, in most of the severe mental illnesses.) Perhaps there is too much dopamine in some brain regions; perhaps the dopamine signal is not being "decoded" properly.

Genetics is another field that is slowly yielding answers to the puzzle of mental illness. Many mental disorders run in families, and studies with twins have borne out suspicions that there is a large genetic component to these diseases.

Nevertheless, researchers now recognize that while inheritance may create a susceptibility, mental illnesses aren't purely genetic in origin. The environment, even within the womb before birth, may also play a role. Environmental stress (the loss of a loved one, job difficulties, and so on, may be important in some mental illnesses), infectious diseases, or other changes in our physical condition may be important in others. All contribute in determining whether a person with a genetic vulnerability will develop a disorder.

There is still much to be learned in these fields; the revolution in brain research has only begun. But I am hopeful that we will soon have the answers to many of our questions about why mental illnesses strike, what effect they have on the brain, and how they can be cured. Already these new discoveries are adding to our understanding of mental illnesses and opening many doors for new treatments. Above all, they tell us that mental illnesses are real illnesses, not moral weaknesses or anyone's fault.

New Treatments Are Saving Lives

Research into new treatments has been as explosive and productive as research into the origins of mental illness. Scientists now have a better understanding of how certain medications affect neurotransmitters in the brain, and their findings have ushered in an era of "designer drugs" with more precise action and fewer unwanted side effects than older medications.

Consider Darrell, who was thirty-seven years old when I met him. He had been in and out of psychiatric hospitals for almost twenty years, suffering from schizophrenia. In between times, he lived on the streets. He had tried one medication after another, but nothing stopped the strange voices he heard. He preached, on the streets and while in the hospital, that his prayers would save the world. In 1989 he had begun treatment with a new drug, clozapine. When I met him, he was greatly improved and about to become a college graduate!

Just a decade ago, there were only a handful of drugs to treat mental illnesses. Sometimes they helped people, sometimes they didn't. Even when they did help, they often caused discouraging side effects. Today, new medications are being developed that are both safer and more effective, even for patients with schizophrenia like Darrell, who had not responded to earlier treatments.

Psychotherapy, popularly known as "talk therapy," and behavior therapy, in which the therapist helps the patient replace negative "habits" with positive behavior, are effective in their own right for certain kinds of symptoms.[3] They are also beneficial when used in association with medication, helping people control undesirable behaviors and develop more constructive ways of dealing with their problems. Brain scans have shown quite dramatically that appropriate psychotherapy can actually change the brain, correcting abnormalities in much the same way that medications do.

These scientific advances are not occurring in a vacuum. Every day I gather evidence of the impact they are having on individuals struggling to overcome their conditions. I receive letters from countless citizens. Many share tales of anguish, but much like Kathy Cronkite, Jerilyn Ross, and Angela Koppenol, others tell of optimism, of newfound health, and of lost lives regained. They offer us hope.

The new treatments reduce symptoms and restore personal effectiveness—not for all patients, but for many; not every time, but quite often; not always permanently, but for long periods of time. Successful treatment for some mental illnesses means that they can be cured; for others it means they can be controlled, and the individuals affected can lead useful, satisfying lives.[4]

Almost everyone, even those with the most persistent and severe disorders, can improve with the new medications and therapy. Yet many who could benefit from treatment are not receiving it. They may be denied access to care because they have no way to pay for it; they may refuse to seek treatment because of the stigma; or they may not even realize that they need medical care or know of the treatment possibilities.

I have learned from my correspondence and from my work over the years, that many sufferers—especially individuals with depression and panic disorder—run from doctor to doctor, thinking that what's bothering them is purely physical. They suffer so much before they finally get help.

Today, when it comes to mental illness, we need to revise our expectations. People need not suffer endlessly in a deteriorating state. As one noted psychiatrist[5] explained, "Not so long ago people with Down's syndrome, a form of mental retardation, were expected to live their lives in institutions. Now this is the exception rather than the norm. Has the nature of the disorder changed? No, what has changed is the vision of what is possible."

In the following chapters, we will look at some of the new breakthroughs in research and treatment that are helping those with mental illness fulfill a new vision, lead more normal lives, and revise our notion of the possibilities.

I have a friend who says, "Illnesses that are understood gain dignity." All of the exciting research you will be reading about is adding to the understanding of mental illnesses that for so long has eluded us. It is my hope that this revolution will endow mental illnesses with a sense of dignity and change the way we regard the people affected by them.

For now, let us take a more detailed look at some of the breakthroughs in particular mental disorders. We'll begin with schizophrenia, since that is the most debilitating and puzzling mental illness of all.

But before we begin, I must warn you that to understand the workings of the brain, you need a Ph.D. in biology—which I don't have! The scientific material about breakthroughs in research is very technical and complex and describing it is not easy. I have tried to simplify the language and make it as easy as possible to comprehend, while still preserving the integrity of the material. It is important for us to have this kind of information so that we can have some idea of what happens in the brain when mental illnesses occur.

Throughout the text I have included definitions of many of the more technical words. For further clarification or information, there is a glossary in the back of the book. The footnotes elaborate on some important but more technical points. Good luck!

The Brain

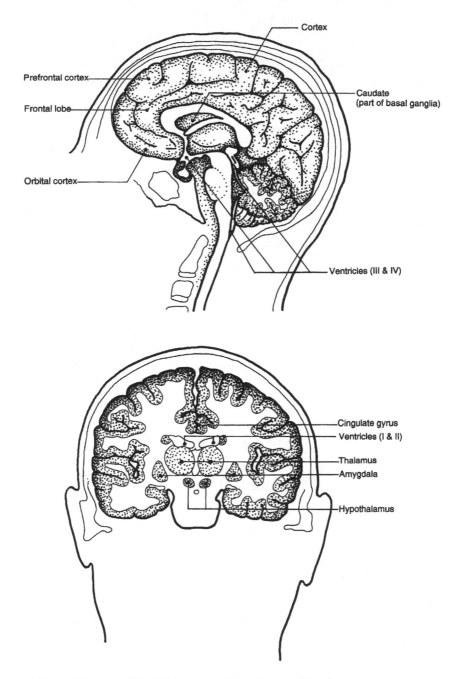

Note: The parts labeled here are those discussed in the text.

Chapter 6

Moving Toward Awakenings: Understanding Schizophrenia

Our understanding of the origins of schizophrenia, which is characterized by disordered thinking, hallucinations, delusions, and a tendency to withdraw from reality, is light-years ahead of what it was just a decade ago. For too long, we blamed faulty parenting for this illness. For too long, we believed that this was a disease that was incomprehensible and intractable. But now, compelling scientific evidence points to the fact that schizophrenia may be caused to a substantial degree by a combination of defects that occur early in the brain's development as a result of genetic vulnerability plus environmental triggers that may be quite physical in nature.

Early Signs

Dr. Elaine Walker is a psychologist at Emory University in Atlanta and the Emory liaison to our mental health program at The Carter Center. She is doing exciting research using an unlikely tool for delving into the mysteries of schizophrenia. She decided to collect childhood home movies of people who had later developed the illness. As these youngsters crawled and toddled, she discovered that they moved their arms and legs and hands in subtly abnormal ways. They splayed their fingers and had odd, jerking, writhing movements. They seemed uncomfortable and irritable and expressed negative emotions such as anger and disgust more frequently than their siblings.

"These are subtle things," she explained to me. "It's not so severe that a parent would say, 'Oh my God, there's something wrong with my child!' But they suggest that the brain abnormalities that create the vulnerability to this devastating illness may be present even at birth."

Others have found that people with schizophrenia are also more likely to have had inexplicable lags and surges in development during infancy and social adjustment and achievement problems as school-age children. Clearly this is a disease that begins early in life, even though the most obvious symptoms do not become apparent until adolescence and early adulthood.

Abnormalities Within the Brain

Much of our new perspective about the origins of schizophrenia comes from the modern imaging techniques. One area of study has been the *cortex,* a major part of the brain's "gray matter" involved in sensing, moving, and thinking. When people with schizophrenia are asked to solve problems that require mental flexibility, PET scans and MRIs show that the *frontal lobes* of the cortex—literally the part of the cortex found in the front of the brain—do not become as active as they do in the brains of people who are well.

There is also evidence that the normally occurring, fluid-filled spaces in the brain (called *ventricles*) are enlarged in schizophrenia patients.[1] Why should the size of the ventricles be significant? Scientists believe that the larger the space, the smaller the total tissue in the brain—thus, less gray matter. This has been confirmed by MRI scans.

Dr. Nancy Andreasen, a psychiatrist at the University of Iowa, points out that the frontal lobes (which constitute nearly 30 percent of the brain) are linked to other key brain structures. Impairment in this area is consistent with many of the symptoms of schizophrenia, including difficulty in processing information, formulating concepts, and organizing thinking and behavior.[2]

An area of the frontal lobes just over the eyes, called the *prefrontal cortex,* has also been implicated in schizophrenia. This is the seat of what is called the "working memory"—our ability to hold new bits of information and interrelate them with what we already know, and to release information we no longer need. It allows us to understand spoken language as well as accomplish tasks in which we must remember visual images that are no longer in view. People with schizophrenia experience a malfunction in this area. They have difficulty clearing their working memory of irrelevant information and keeping visual images in mind after they have disappeared from sight.[3]

Other sites in the brain where abnormalities seem to occur in this illness include an area called the *thalamus,* which helps us filter, process, and relay input from our senses, emotions, and memory. According to Dr. Andreasen, "a person with a defective thalamus is likely to be flooded with information and overwhelmed with stimuli." She found that the thalamus is, on average, smaller in people with schizophrenia than in the rest of the population.

Taken together, these many defects make it difficult for the various parts of the brain to communicate with one another. They bring about a failure in the memory and information processing mechanisms within the brain.

What causes these problems? Studies show that the miswiring of *neurons* (brain cells) can occur around the fourth to sixth month of pregnancy when the brain is organizing itself and neurons are settling into their proper places and when the entire cortex is growing rapidly.[4]

A dietary deficiency (including severe malnutrition) or an attack of influenza or some other viral infection of the pregnant mother might interfere with this process and cause these various defects in brain circuitry and architecture in a child who is genetically vulnerable.[5] The viral infection theory is based on the discovery of *antibodies* (molecules the body manufactures to protect itself against invaders such as viruses and bacteria) that are specific to the brain in the blood of people with schizophrenia. Also, abnormal proteins linked to a herpesvirus that strikes the brain have been found in the fluid surrounding the spinal cord in 30 percent of people with schizophrenia. These proteins do not exist in mentally healthy individuals. It is likely that some of these viral infections occurred prenatally.

Oxygen deprivation during development in the womb may also play a role. This can be caused by the umbilical cord wrapping around the neck of the fetus or the mother's placenta being torn or compressed. The higher the number of oxygen-related complications during pregnancy, the greater one's chances of developing schizophrenia.[6]

Sometimes scientists have a personal reason for becoming interested in researching a particular illness. Meggin Hollister, clinical psychologist at the University of Pennsylvania, is one of these—her sister Annick suffers from schizophrenia. Dr. Hollister has found that children whose Rh factor differs from their mother's might have a greater chance of developing the disease. This makes the fetus vulnerable to attack by its mother's immune system and can cause permanent neurological damage.[7]

Any or all of these prenatal events could have triggered the brain abnormalities that the new brain-scanning technology has identified.

Another interesting area of inquiry relates to the fact that the brains of people with schizophrenia have too much dopamine (the neurotransmitter mentioned earlier), which regulates movement and influences mood and motivation. In the 1940s and 50s, it was discovered that drugs like amphetamines and cocaine sometimes created symptoms in healthy people similar to schizophrenia and temporarily worsened symptoms in those who were already ill. Later it was found that these drugs had their effect by increasing neurotransmitters such as dopamine in the brain. New medications seemed to work because they blocked the dopamine receptors.[8] Although it is still unclear how dopamine and its receptors influence schizophrenia, it seems evident that they do play an important role in the disease.

There is also strong evidence that schizophrenia runs in families. In numerous studies of fraternal and identical twins, it has been found that in nearly 50 percent of identical twins (who have exactly the same genes), both children became ill, while both twins became ill in less than 4 percent of fraternal twins (who have only some genes in common). And adopted children whose biological parents have schizophrenia are much more likely to develop the illness than those whose biological parents do not.[9]

However, the genetics of this disease are complex. What is inherited is not the disease itself but a predisposition for developing it, much like inheriting a risk for diabetes or heart disease. The genes (and many genes are certainly involved) set the stage so that an environmental "insult" such as low oxygen or a viral infection in the womb might lead to the defects in brain development that produce schizophrenia.

Because its origins and manifestations can be so diverse, experts have speculated that schizophrenia is perhaps not one disease at all, but several related conditions that have been collected under one catchall diagnosis.

No matter what the cause, somehow the brain of a person afflicted with this disease did not form the connections that humans normally require. Many teams of scientists are hard at work identifying the whys and wherefores of all of those disruptions, and they are making good progress. Let's look at some of their accomplishments.

A Revolution in Treatment

Dramatic progress has been made in the treatment of schizophrenia in the last decade. Antipsychotic drugs to treat the illness have multiplied.[10] And though there is still no cure, these new medications help reduce symptoms and offer hope for a longer, happier life.

Traditional antipsychotic medications for schizophrenia, prescribed since the early 1950s, are called *neuroleptics.* They have been effective in suppressing the hallucinations, delusions, and disorganized thinking of schizophrenia (the "positive symptoms"). Their discovery heralded the end of "treatment by physical restraint" in the dark days before reform.

Thorazine is one of the best known of these neuroleptics. Originally developed as an antihistamine, a chance observation that it had some antipsychotic properties led to its use in schizophrenia. Once it was established that it helped reduce symptoms, scientists sought to discover why. They found that Thorazine works on the dopamine system, decreasing the amount and overactivity of dopamine in the brain—the presumed cause of the positive symptoms.

Unfortunately, the neuroleptics are not effective in relieving the "negative symptoms" of schizophrenia—lack of interest in activities and people, decreased motivation and self-care, reduced ability for communication and emotional expression. These symptoms can be extremely disabling since they tend to result in withdrawal and social isolation.

Moreover, many patients do not respond to the neuroleptic medications, or, if they do, they usually suffer disturbing side effects including muscle spasms, Parkinson's-like tremors, stiff gait, slowed speech, and sexual dysfunction. The most serious side effect is tardive dyskinesia (TD), a dreadful condition, sometimes irreversible, in which a person experiences repetitive involuntary movements, such as lip-smacking, facial grimacing, and abnormal gestures. It develops late in treatment, usually after several years. Despite the benefits of neuroleptics, these side effects (and the side effects of medications given to counteract them) often leave patients with a great deal of mental and physical impairment.[11]

Newer antipsychotic medications are being developed in an effort to better treat the negative symptoms of schizophrenia and reduce the side effects. Clozapine (sold as Clozaril), which my acquaintance, Darrell, is taking, is the first of this new class and is effective for at least a third of those patients who have not responded to traditional medications.[12] Equally important, it helps to ameliorate both the negative and the positive symptoms of the illness[13]—perhaps a first for an antipsychotic medication—with fewer side effects and no risk of causing tardive dyskinesia. It does have one serious drawback: it can produce a life-threatening blood disorder in 1 to 2 percent of patients.[14] When it is given, blood counts must be checked regularly to prevent this terrible side effect.

For some patients this medication seems even to have the power to restore a semblance of the "lost self"—the personality of the individual before the symptoms took hold. In a recent mental health journal dedicated to the "awakenings" that can happen following treatment with clozapine, one patient was described this way: "It was as if the psychotic stranger had disappeared and the pentimento of the real self had reemerged."[15]

The success of clozapine, by providing marked relief without the terrible side effects (which it had been assumed that all antipsychotic drugs would have), has led to what has been called a renaissance in the search for drugs to treat schizophrenia. It has encouraged researchers to design new and even more effective drugs that target specific areas of the brain while avoiding others.

One such drug, introduced in 1996, is risperidone (Risperdal). It is currently the most widely prescribed medication for schizophrenia in the nation. Risperidone has similar effects as clozapine on symptoms without the danger of developing the blood disorder.[16] Unfortunately, it is not quite as good as clozapine in treating negative symptoms.

A sixty-five-year-old woman with schizoaffective disorder (a mental condition involving symptoms of both schizophrenia and mood disorders) described her condition after two years on risperidone:

> My thinking has become more and more logical. . . . My dreams and goals are more realistic, rather than fantasy-based and childlike. I accept that I have choices, and instead of being a victim, I make choices. . . . My ability to think about my past, present and future is the result of Risperdal enhancing my brain activity. . . . The longer I am on it, the better my brain reacts. . . . My mind is quieter and easier to be with, now. Without the din, I can recognize the needs of my body and I am more able to care for myself. . . . I feel like a regular person. In fact, I am a regular person with regular feelings and desires. I no longer think of myself as a mental patient.[17]

Although these medications represent a major step forward in the treatment of schizophrenia, there are other promising new medications on the horizon that may prove to be even safer and more effective. Olanzapine (Zyprexa) may affect more areas of the brain than either clozapine or risperidone while having fewer side effects. It was introduced in late 1996. During my recent visit to NIMH, I met two people with schizophrenia who, as a part of a research study, were being treated with this medication: Latasha, a pretty African-American woman in her late teens, who had only been ill for six months; and Ron, a man of about thirty-five or forty, who had been ill for some time. Ron held a college degree and had worked in the community before becoming ill. He had a slight tremor in his hands, a remnant of his treatment with an older neuroleptic.

"Ron had severe tremors when he came here," his physician explained, "but we took him off other medications and changed him to Zyprexa. And though it's still a bit early to tell, he seems to be doing much better now."

I was proud of Latasha and Ron and told them so. "What you are doing is really important. By being willing to come into this hospital to try new treatments, you may be helping yourself, but you may also be helping many, many other people."

What they are doing *is* really important. The researchers at NIMH always need people who are willing to join in clinical trials. This is the only way to test the effectiveness of new medications and treatments. I was informed later that both Latasha and Ron improved with the new medication, and both have been dismissed from the research program.

Many more drugs, all of which have the potential to significantly improve the quality of life of countless individuals with schizophrenia, are still in the research pipeline. Yet medications are not the whole answer to the treatment of this disease.

Awakenings

Many professionals describe the "awakenings" that their patients experience once they begin these medications. They liken the new and sudden return to this world with Rip Van Winkle's experience—but often sadder.

Some individuals drop out of treatment because they find it difficult to give up the psychotic personality they have lived with for so long. Dane Wingerson, a psychiatrist in Seattle, Washington, described how one of his patients, Henry, had believed himself to be God while suffering from schizophrenia. After two weeks on one of the new antipsychotic drugs, he refused further treatment with the explanation "It's tough not being God anymore."

"Prior to the new medication," Dr. Wingerson explained, "Henry had a very important job that took up all of his time. He felt important and respected. It didn't matter that he had no friends and that he lived in a rundown apartment. I guess when you're God you can live just as you please. But the new medication changed all that. Henry was no longer psychotic, and he woke up to find that he was profoundly alone, in his mid-forties in a very different world that perplexed and frightened him. All he seemed to have to look forward to was his rundown digs, his monthly SSI survival bucks, the two packs of cigarettes a day."[18]

Dr. Wingerson's experience with Henry underscores the importance of psychotherapy and family support for individuals who are emerging from psychotic states as a result of the new treatments. Indeed, depression and suicide are serious threats when awakening schizophrenia patients realize that they have lost so many years of their lives. Because the illness reaches its full form during adolescence and early adulthood, many have missed crucial developmental and educational milestones—how to make small talk and ask someone for a date, how to apply for and hold down a job, how to study and write a term paper. Consequently, they find readjustment to be hard work.

Group counseling with peers has been found to be particularly helpful in offering support and readjustment into social life for these individuals who are reconnecting to their lost selves. Therapy, whether group or individual, can help them reconstruct their personalities and regain self-esteem.[19] While psychotherapy alone cannot "cure" schizophrenia, it can play a critical role in improving an individual's functioning, social skills, quality of life, and motivation to stay on the medication. Family therapy is also important.[20]

Though Henry could not readjust to normalcy, Sam, another of Dr. Wingerson's patients, did well on the new medication—aided by the loving support of his family. Sam had tried the older neuroleptics but stopped taking them on several occasions because he couldn't tolerate the side effects. Once on the new medication, he was able to work part- and then full-time in a convenience store his brother managed. He interacted well with the public, made a few friends, and moved out of his mother's home to live independently with an older brother.

After his initial inpatient phase of treatment, Sam's mother and sister had worked closely with him to make sure he took his medication and helped him "look forward to a different type of future." They persuaded his brother to give him the job. They called him frequently and invited him for meals. "I don't need angels anymore," Sam told Dr. Wingerson recently. "I've got my family."

"Medications may be a cornerstone of treatment," Dr. Wingerson concluded, "but treatment cannot be successful unless all dimensions of an affected individual's life are addressed and supported. To be psychosis free with nothing to look forward to can be devastating."[21]

Although there are no definite explanations for the exact causes of this disorder, the exciting news is that even schizophrenia is slowly yielding up its secrets. And as scientists continue their discoveries and as better and better therapies are forthcoming, there is very real optimism in the mental health community for those afflicted and for their families and friends. Dan Weisburd, publisher of the journal of the California Alliance for the Mentally Ill, puts it this way: "Hope has awakened and you can almost touch it."

Chapter 7

Taming the Black Dog: Understanding Depression

What would cause highly successful people like Rod Steiger, Kathy Cronkite, and even television reporter Mike Wallace and British prime minister Sir Winston Churchill to develop depression, a mood disorder characterized by feelings of sadness, dejection, and despair? Churchill referred to his illness as a "black dog." As with schizophrenia, the exact causes of this illness have not yet been determined, though scientists theorize that all mental illnesses may be the result of several interrelated factors.

Major depression seems to occur in some families generation after generation, indicating that heredity may play an important role in a person's vulnerability to the illness. Research has shown that if one identical twin has manic-depression, the other has a 70 percent chance of developing it. In addition, a child adopted into a family in which someone is suffering from depression has no greater chance of developing the illness than the general rates in the population.[1]

However, depression can also occur in people who have no family history of the illness. As in diseases like diabetes, where vulnerability depends on more than one gene and where environmental factors matter, depression may "skip a generation."

People with low self-esteem, who consistently view themselves and the world with pessimism, or who are readily overwhelmed by stress are prone to depression. Very often, it is the genetic vulnerability combined with life experiences that bring on the illness.

Stress, often in the form of a personal loss, can trigger a first episode of depression in someone who is genetically vulnerable. This loss could include being laid off from one's job, a divorce, an unwelcome retirement, natural disasters, legal problems, a physical assault (as in the case of Angela Koppenol I described in chapter 1), or the death of a loved one. Later episodes may develop without such an event, and if one is repeatedly exposed to stress, it can cause the episodes to occur more frequently.

The loss of a parent during childhood is a particularly distressing event that can pave the way for depression later in life. Chronic, long-term illness can also be a stressor. Depression can occur along with and as a result of a stroke, heart attack, or cancer. A January 17, 1996, *New York Times* article reported that depression has been diagnosed in 50 percent of patients who were hospitalized for strokes; six months later, 90 percent of those individuals were still depressed.[2]

How does stress trigger depression? Researchers have found that upsetting situations arouse a part of the brain called the *amygdala,* a small, almond-shaped region that recognizes and regulates emotions, especially fear and anger, and another region at the very base of the brain called the *hypothalamus.* If these brain regions overreact to stress, perhaps because of a genetic vulnerability, they may produce a chemical chain reaction that leads to depression.[3]

In fact, researchers believe that decreased amounts of serotonin and other neurotransmitters are involved in depression, causing the sleep problems, irritability, anxiety, fatigue, and despondent mood that characterize the illness.[4]

Decreased serotonin activity may be linked to suicidal behavior, according to psychiatrist Jonathan Mann at Columbia University. Autopsies of suicide victims have revealed lesser amounts of serotonin in the fluid surrounding the brain and spinal cord than is normal, and certain brain cells[5] in these victims seem to have more receptors for serotonin, as if to make up for the inadequate supply.

MRI and PET scans have also revealed decreased activity in an area of the prefrontal cortex (see diagram on page 130) of individuals with depression. This area has been found to be much smaller than average in individuals who suffer from depression and bipolar illness, although it is still unclear whether this abnormality is the cause or consequence of the illness.[6] Not surprisingly, scientists believe that it is not just decreased activity in one area of the brain that influences mood disorders, but that other structures are also involved.[7]

It is interesting how research sometimes takes unexpected turns. Depression expert Dr. Mark S. Gold reports that sleep-wake patterns in depressed individuals seem to run "backwards."[8] The normal sleep pattern is made up of several ninety-minute cycles during the night with various stages of deeper sleep plus REM (rapid eye movement) sleep—an almost waking state in which dreams occur. For most of us, deep sleep occurs early in the night, with REM sleep being only a small fraction of the first ninety-minute cycle and taking up more time in the cycles as the night progresses.

The pattern seems to reverse for depressed individuals. They experience long stretches of the more wakeful REM sleep early in the night, less toward morning. This sleep pattern may account for some of the exhaustion many depressed people feel when they wake up. These findings support the view that depression arises from a disturbance in one's biological clock.

Some researchers are also investigating the relationship between sunlight and depression. Individuals afflicted with *seasonal affective disorder (SAD)*—a form of depression—become gloomy as nights become longer. As if getting ready to hibernate for the winter, they crave carbohydrates and become lethargic. They oversleep, gain weight, and feel generally fatigued during fall and winter months.

Dr. Norman E. Rosenthal of the National Institute of Mental Health in Bethesda,[9] one of the first to identify SAD as an illness, explains that light and latitude have much to do with this type of depression. "Somebody here in Maryland," he says, "who might have had bad seasonal affective disorder might have been disabled when she went up to Toronto and might have felt much better the few years that she lived in Florida and might have been completely cured in Guam."

Scientists now believe that SAD is related to how much light is hitting the retina of the eye. The less light, the more of a natural sleep hormone is circulating in the body. In scientific experiments, when lab animals were injected with this hormone they overate, overslept, and became lethargic.[10]

Depressed people also experience abnormalities in hormones that affect appetite and sex drive. In women, hormonal imbalances related to menstruation, pregnancy, childbirth, and menopause have been related to depression. These findings suggest that our hormones may also be regulated by the neurotransmitters that regulate our moods.

In some individuals, depression takes a milder but more extended form called *dysthymia,* which is characterized by a continual sense of sadness that can last for years. The long duration of this state can seriously wear people down. Those affected cannot function up to their potential. They are also vulnerable to superimposed major depressive episodes.

⁂

When Rod Steiger stated, "I have a clinical depression, which is a chemical imbalance of the brain," at our Conversations at The Carter Center, he knew what he was talking about.

Let's see how the new so-called designer drugs are now successfully adjusting brain chemistry so that depression is no longer the scourge it once was.

Treatments: More Effective Than Ever

A few years ago, a friend of ours, a well-respected businessman, was suffering from depression, but he didn't know it. One day, on a chance meeting, he asked if I had time for a cup of coffee. He actually was helping me with one of my projects, and I just assumed that he wanted to talk about it. The conversation began normally with small talk. Then he said, "I may not be able to do that work for you. I have some serious problems."

I was surprised; Fred had always been rather reserved and we had never discussed personal matters. But with eyes averted, he continued, "I don't know what's the matter with me. I can't concentrate. I don't want to do anything; my work is suffering; my family life is suffering; all I want to do is lie around in the daytime, and I can't remember a night when I've slept. I'm just not good for anything or anybody anymore." He was embarrassed, and he was scared. He thought he might have cancer or another serious illness, but none of the doctors he consulted could find anything wrong with him.

Although he said he was confiding in me because he felt guilty about not having finished the work he had promised, I knew that he was aware of my interest in mental health. I suspected that he was worried about a mental problem but didn't want to admit it. He was obviously relieved when I told him this was not unusual, that it happened to many people, and that I was sure he could get help. I recommended a psychiatrist, and he went to see him immediately. He had worried and suffered so long that he was ready to do anything, even if it meant a diagnosis of mental illness.

The psychiatrist concluded that Fred suffered from depression and prescribed an antidepressant medication. He actually prescribed a number of them before he hit on the right one. Within weeks, Fred was feeling better and was able to get back to his normal activities. Today, he is perfectly fine: His business is prospering and his marriage is intact.

Many people think that if they have a single episode of mental illness, they will be mentally ill forever. But when someone is depressed and gets help, the illness doesn't necessarily return. Although it may become chronic if untreated, the good news is that for many people, depression may not recur when properly treated. Some people need to stay on their medication for a long time; others don't. Some can benefit from psychotherapy alone; others require therapy and medication.

Indeed, the most common and effective treatment for severely depressed individuals is a combination of psychotherapy and antidepressant medication. These two approaches reinforce each other—the psychotherapy puts those affected in a frame of mind that makes them more apt to stick to their medication schedule, and the medication puts them in the frame of mind that makes their therapy more beneficial.

Whatever the course of treatment, PET scans have confirmed that effective psychotherapy and medical treatment are associated with a normalization of the area of the brain (prefrontal cortex) that shows decreased activity in depressed individuals.[11]

Drug Therapies

Many myths have swirled around the use of antidepressants—that they are addictive, that they are uppers, that they rob one of independence. Perhaps these misconceptions have sprung from the way depression was treated in the 1950s and 60s—with habit-forming tranquilizers such as Valium that masked symptoms rather than treating them. But today's antidepressants are neither tranquilizers, nor "uppers," nor addictive. They are a distinct group of medications that work specifically on brain chemistry.

Treatment with antidepressant medications has helped millions of people overcome major depression.[12] They have been approved for adults, the elderly, and even children.

And as my friend Fred discovered, there are many of these antidepressants available, and there is no way to predict which one will be most effective—some individuals respond well to one drug but not at all to another. Each person is unique and must be evaluated and treated as such. The doctor may proceed by trial and error until a satisfactory treatment is found. Sometimes complex blood tests are performed to detect neurotransmitters, enzymes, and hormones associated with the illness in order to identify the proper medication with as little delay as possible.

Once treatment begins, usually the first sign that the medication is working appears in two to three weeks as the insomnia, a major symptom of depression, begins to abate. The other symptoms usually diminish over the next several weeks.[13]

As depressed individuals begin to feel better, they may think they no longer need their medication. This is a mistake. It is vital to take the antidepressant regularly, not just when feeling depressed. The drug's effectiveness depends upon its regular use and the consistent levels of the medication in the blood. Even after the depression lifts, the physician may keep the patient on the drug for four to twelve months or longer, to prevent relapse. At that point, the doctor may slowly eliminate the medication without the patient relapsing.

There are several different classes of antidepressant medications that are most often used to treat depression. Each of these medications acts to keep one or another of the brain chemicals (neurotransmitters) in balance. The newer class called selective serotonin reuptake inhibitors, or SSRIs, which includes Prozac, Zoloft, and Paxil, among others, has been hailed as a breakthrough in the treatment of depression. Above all, they cause fewer side effects than older antidepressants. In addition, since they seem to interact less with many other medications, they can be safely prescribed for elderly patients who may be suffering from other medical conditions that require drug therapy.[14]

Nevertheless, side effects can occur even with SSRIs. These may include insomnia, drowsiness, headache, nausea, constipation, or decreased sexual desire. These side effects, though, can be minimal. And if an individual feels uncomfortable with one medication, others may be just as effective, or even more so, without the discomfort. Anyone experiencing side effects should report them to his or her doctor. See appendix C for a more detailed description.

Psychotherapy

Psychotherapy is used alone to treat mild to moderate depression and in combination with medications for severe depression.

The therapist using this type of treatment may help a depressed individual focus on pessimistic, self-defeating, automatic thoughts. The thought could be, I'm a failure, and I will never succeed. By asking questions such as "Are you a failure in every situation or is there one situation in which you didn't fail in the last day, week, or month?" the negative thoughts are challenged. When they can be recognized and dispelled, the depressed person's mood improves.

Sometimes, patients may be encouraged to bring up memories of long-repressed conflicts in order to work through them with an empathetic therapist. This can help them better understand themselves; in turn, they feel better about themselves and the depression lifts.

It is important to recognize that therapy can often be a two-steps-forward-one-step-back process. Sometimes healing comes in tiny steps, but it is healing, nonetheless.

Behavior Therapy

Whereas psychotherapy focuses on changing thoughts, behavior therapy focuses on replacing negative "habits" with positive behavior. While homework plays an important role in this type of therapy, patients are also encouraged to renew their social lives and take part in activities that they once enjoyed. This may be difficult at first, but it can help lift the depression, or at least break the cycle of lethargy and fatigue.

Psychotherapy and behavior therapy have been found to be helpful for one third to one half of those treated, but since both require active participation, these therapies may not be a good "fit," at least not initially, for those who are severely depressed.

Electroconvulsive Therapy (ECT)

Many of us have terrible visions of torture chambers when we imagine someone receiving electroconvulsive therapy, formerly known as shock therapy. Fortunately, dramatic improvements have been made in these treatments, and today they are performed in a carefully controlled manner. They are given only after an individual has been sedated with a short-acting anesthetic and a muscle relaxant. Patients neither remember nor feel the treatment.

Usually, six to twelve treatments are given in intervals of two to three days. The mild electrical current used seems to affect the part of the brain that regulates mood and helps stimulate the chemicals that are in such short supply in depressed individuals. There can be a brief period of memory loss and confusion following treatment, but usually this ameliorates within a short period of time.

ECT is still used as a last resort, although psychiatrists John H. Greist and James W. Jefferson write in their book, *Depression and Its Treatment,* "A new technique called brief-pulse ECT uses the minimum amount of electricity needed to produce an effective treatment and substantially reduces memory loss after each treatment and over a course of treatments."[15]

It's appropriate to consider ECT for patients with severe depression who have not responded to several medications. It has proven to be highly effective and fast-acting in these cases.

Recently, a friend of ours was severely depressed during a serious illness. No medication seemed to snap him out of it. One day we learned that he had undergone ECT, and we were very concerned . . . until the physician reassured us, explaining the great improvements in the treatment. Sure enough, our friend's depression lifted immediately, and he became his old self again.

ECT may also be beneficial for an individual who has made a serious suicide attempt or for the depressed individual who becomes psychotic. In addition, someone who suffers from other medical illnesses may be unable to participate in psychotherapy or tolerate antidepressant medication, but he or she can receive this treatment effectively.

It is important to note that little research has been done to establish the effectiveness of ECT beyond the short term. Also, available evidence suggests that relapse rates in the year follow-ing the treatment are likely to be high unless the patient takes maintenance antidepressant medications.

❧

Depression is the most treatable of all the mental illnesses. With our new knowledge of the brain, diagnoses are more accurate and treatments have improved considerably, bringing relief to many who have suffered. If you or someone you care about is having symptoms that you think may be the result of depres-sion, you should seek help from a mental health professional. There is no need to suffer unnecessarily when there is so much help available.

Chapter 8

A Life Worth Living:
Understanding Manic-Depression

In April 1996, the National Institute of Mental Health announced that scientists were closing in on five separate gene sites for manic-depressive or bipolar illness, which involves cycles of depression alternating with elation or mania. Dr. Edward Ginns,[1] a key investigator in this research, said, "These findings suggest a complex mode of inheritance, similar to that seen in diseases like diabetes and hypertension.

"An individual's risk for developing bipolar disorder probably increases with each susceptible gene carried," he explained. "Inheriting one gene is probably not sufficient." Dr. Ginns based these findings on investigations of seventeen families of an Old Amish order that have an unusually high incidence of manic-depression. They all trace their ancestry back to a single eighteenth-century pioneer family that suffered from the illness.

This research underscores the important role genetics may play in one's vulnerability to manic-depressive illness.[2] In fact, it has been found that between 80 and 90 percent of those afflicted have relatives who have some type of depression. But people with a genetic predisposition do not always develop the illness. As with other mental illnesses, environmental factors play a role in determining the onset.

Genetic factors, though, are the most clearly established biological findings about manic-depressive illness, and they set the
stage for the disorder. Because many people who suffer from
manic-depression respond to medication that alters brain chemistry, it appears that this illness is also caused, at least in part, by
an imbalance in neurotransmitters and, as with other mental illnesses, by certain abnormalities in the brain.

Studies have found higher levels of stress hormones in people
with bipolar illness. And as mentioned in chapter 7, a specific
area in the prefrontal cortex is smaller in individuals with bipolar
illness than in people who are not afflicted with this disorder.[3]

Perhaps one's genetic heritage leads to abnormalities in the
brain that might cause these imbalances when triggered by
stress. Further investigation is still needed to find all the answers.

Medications

The recent Ann Landers column mentioned in chapter 5
echoed so many letters I receive from citizens every day:

> About seven months ago, I was a highly regarded vice
> president of a large company. Overnight, I developed an
> obnoxious personality, becoming pushy, arrogant, and
> disruptive. My behavior was a major topic of company
> gossip as co-workers talked about the radical change in
> my demeanor. One day, I lost my temper and yelled at
> the chairman of the board. I was promptly fired.
>
> Over the next few months, my mental state deterio-
> rated to the point where I would sit in front of the TV
> and argue with the news anchor. I believed an asteroid
> was going to hit earth. I was nonfunctional and finally
> hospitalized.

It was then I discovered that I had a chemical imbalance in my brain that caused a medical condition known as bipolar disorder. This is easily treated with lithium. After a few months, I felt like myself again.[4]

Lithium has been a godsend for many with bipolar illness. Braxton, my neighbor with the illness, is taking lithium to control his symptoms. In fact, this mood-stabilizing medication is the most commonly prescribed for those diagnosed with manic-depressive disorder. For many people, it is effective in treating both the depressive and manic phases of the illness and in preventing recurrences, but it must be taken regularly. Its effectiveness will be lost by stopping the medication and then restarting it during a manic episode.[5]

Side effects of lithium can include excessive thirst, urinary problems, lack of coordination, tremors, nausea and vomiting, and fatigue. Because of these side effects, and for the sake of the 30 to 40 percent of sufferers who are not helped by the drug, scientists are continuing to work on new treatments.

One such medication, the anticonvulsive Depakote, was approved for the treatment of acute mania in 1996. It is the first drug since lithium's introduction in the late 1960s to be endorsed by the Food and Drug Administration for the treatment of manic-depression. Other anticonvulsants, including divalproex and Tegretil, has recently been found to be effective in treating mania, too. And clozapine and risperidone, drugs normally used to treat schizophrenia, are also being prescribed for mania and psychosis in combination with other mood-stabilizing medications. These drugs can dramatically improve the lives of people suffering from bipolar disorder, although there is no cure yet for the illness.

Psychotherapy is highly recommended for treating manic-depression but is helpful only in conjunction with medication.

In her fascinating book *An Unquiet Mind,* Dr. Kay Redfield Jamison,[6] a professor of psychiatry with manic-depression herself, describes how helpful her therapist was to her recovery after a suicide attempt:

> The debt I owe my psychiatrist is beyond description. I remember sitting in his office a hundred times during those grim months and each time thinking, What on earth can he say that will make me feel better or keep me alive? Well, there never was anything he could say, that's the funny thing. It was all the stupid, desperately optimistic, condescending things he didn't say that kept me alive; all the compassion and warmth I felt from him that could not have been said; all the intelligence, competence, and time he put into it; and his granite belief that mine was a life worth living. . . . He taught me that the road from suicide to life is cold and colder and colder still, but—with steely effort, the grace of God, and an inevitable break in the weather—that I could make it.[7]

As a professor of psychiatry, Dr. Jamison teaches medical residents and interns about the illness she struggled with herself. "My own experience as a patient," she writes, "had made me particularly aware of how critical psychotherapy could be in making sense of the pain; how it could keep me alive long enough to have a chance at getting well; and how it could help one to learn to reconcile the resentments at taking medication with the terrible consequences of not taking it."[8]

Family therapy is particularly important in the treatment of bipolar illness. In one recent study,[9] patients whose families participated in eighteen therapy sessions had higher recovery rates and were half as likely to be rehospitalized for their illness two years later as those whose families did not participate. The therapy focused on family communication and problem-solving. All family members learned how to respond to their ill loved ones more effectively, especially when they were in a manic phase. In addition, the therapy seemed to help patients keep to their medication schedules, reduced stress, and enabled family members to be more supportive.

Susan Swedo,[10] acting scientific director of the National Institute of Mental Health, confirms the importance of family involvement. She writes, "With bipolar disorder . . . the efforts of each member of the team [the family, the patient, and the psychiatrist] are needed to help identify the early warning signs of a manic episode, since the patient may be less willing or able to seek help when she is experiencing the pleasurable effects of hypomania [a severe form of mania] . . . or the poor judgment of a full-blown manic episode. It is equally important to identify the signals of an approaching depressive episode, since the patient is most vulnerable to despair during the 'switch' between mania and depression. The team must also work together to ensure that the patient takes her medication exactly as prescribed, even during times when she feels well, in order to prevent recurrences. Manic-depression is clearly a chronic illness, and ongoing monitoring and assessment are essential."

It is not as widely appreciated as it should be that most affective disorders such as depression and manic-depression can be treated successfully. For example, under optimal treatment with the drug lithium, persons with manic-depressive illness live an average of seven years longer than those not receiving treatment, and experience nine to ten years of more normal health and effective functioning, years that would otherwise have been lost to the illness.

Over the past several decades, these disorders have served as a principal focus for scientific research, and the results have literally been life-saving. Thirty years ago, one in every five patients with manic-depressive illness died by suicide, as did countless numbers of people who had depression. Today, lithium, antidepressant medications, anticonvulsants, ECT, and supportive psychosocial treatments are effective for most, though not all, people suffering from depressive disorders. And although significant progress has been made, researchers are striving to discover still more effective treatments for these debilitating disorders.

Chapter 9

Raising the Threshold: Understanding Anxiety Disorders

As with the other brain diseases we have examined, when we talk about the origins of anxiety disorders, we are dealing with the issues of vulnerability and environment. "We know the predisposition to these disorders runs in families," explained Jerilyn Ross, a former sufferer of panic attacks and founder of the Anxiety Disorders Association of America. "We know there's a genetic component, although the exact nature of the disorder and the specific symptoms do not necessarily manifest themselves in the same way amongst family members. We know that there are biological causes, and psychological and environmental triggers.

"A lot of people will have their first panic attack after there has been a separation or change in their life or a major loss like a death of a loved one. I like to think of it as something being 'off' in the wiring of the brain," she continued. "There's a different threshold for panic. One of the ways I explain it to people is to have them imagine that suddenly there's an earthquake. Your heart is pounding, you're sweaty, you want to run, you want to hide. That's a normal, natural protective response our body has. Biologically, we go into the 'fight or flight' response.

"But for some of us, there's something in our body chemistry that triggers the alarm for no reason. It's a beautiful day. You're sitting here and all of a sudden, you have a sensation, your brain is getting the message of danger, trouble, fight, run, hide, get out, and all the physiological things that go with it. So it's really a normal reaction but it's happening at the wrong time."

I questioned Jerilyn about the stress that precipitated her first attack, which I described in chapter 2—after all, the scene at the music festival that she had described in Salzburg seemed so exquisite. She explained that the body cannot judge between good stress and bad stress. "It was almost like a sensory overload," she replied. "It was an awesome evening, and it kicked something in. Once you have that biological event the first time . . ." She paused for a moment as if to consider her words. "You can have one panic attack in your life and the rest of your life be haunted by it. It's such a profound event."

Some researchers have found that the propensity for anxiety disorders may begin in childhood. Rachel Gittleman Klein, director of psychology at New York State Psychiatric Institute, notes that some people who later develop these disorders experienced intense separation anxiety as children.[1] That model fit Jerilyn Ross. "I was classic," Jerilyn explained. "I once ripped my mother's skirt off on the street because she tried to get me to go to school. I wouldn't go to camp, I wouldn't stay at friends' houses."

New Insights into the Causes

In December 1996, it was announced with great fanfare that people who had a variation in one particular gene had a tendency to be more anxiety-prone than those who did not. It was believed that this gene subtly influenced how the brain uses serotonin. Less than six months later, another group of scientists declared there was no such correlation—at least in the population they tested.

Scientific investigation is filled with many debates, controversies, and obstacles, especially when it comes to the field of neuroscience, where there is so much left to be discovered. But this is most certainly part of the research process and is the way we make progress in both identifying causes and improving treatment.

Anxiety is a normal human emotion with which we are all familiar, but it can become extreme, leading to panic disorders, phobias, or other illnesses. What do we know about the origins of these anxiety disorders? Are there areas in the brain associated with them? What about genetic links? Most of the current research has focused on panic disorder and obsessive-compulsive disorder, so I will explore these with you.

Panic Disorder

Several theories have been set forth to explain panic disorder. One suggests that some individuals overreact to the sweaty palms and racing heart that appear as the first sign of anxiety. They misinterpret these as signs of a heart attack or some other catastrophe, and they become more and more afraid until the anxiety escalates into full-blown panic. These hypersensitive individuals have a profound reaction to symptoms that others are able to dismiss as merely unpleasant or annoying.

As with most mental illnesses, scientists have now learned that genetics, brain chemicals (neurotransmitters), and brain structures all seem to play a role in panic disorder. Higher rates of panic disorder have been found among parents and siblings of those with the illness, implicating genetics. And since medications that act on serotonin and certain other neurotransmitters help to control panic attacks, scientists believe that these neurotransmitters are somehow associated with the disorder. In fact, a number of people with depression, which can also be treated by medications that act on serotonin, also have panic disorder. This has suggested that the causes of both of these illnesses may be related in the brain. Of course, panic disorder can be helped by anti-anxiety medications that do not help depression, so there are also important differences.

As for brain structures, research suggests that there are nerve cells programmed to recognize danger, releasing chemicals that cause us to have feelings of anxiety and fear.[2] But in the case of anxiety disorders, these feelings may be too strong (panic) and may come even when no real danger is present.

The amygdala, the almond-shaped brain structure that we learned might contribute to depression (see chapter 7), is involved in deciding whether a noise or a sight we experience is worthy of a fearful reaction.[3] This is important to protect us from truly dangerous situations. Usually, the amygdala makes a split-second determination and moves on to monitoring the next experience. The theory is that in panic disorder, the amygdala responds powerfully to false alarms or becomes fixated on a stimulus—such as finding oneself on a high floor without an easy way down—and doesn't move on. It repeatedly tells the rest of the brain there is something grave to fear, causing it to release a deluge of neurotransmitters. These then produce a rapid heartbeat, sweating, dizziness, churning stomach, and so on.

Treatments for Panic Disorder

In her book *Triumph over Fear,* Jerilyn Ross describes the debates that raged in the 1980s among those who advocated medications for panic disorder versus those who believed psychotherapy was the only reasonable treatment. Polarities were established between nature and nurture, biology and psychology.

"Seemingly overnight, the debates became virtual love feasts," she writes. "What happened was the astonishing discovery that not only did both approaches work, but used together they were synergistic—that is, drug therapy plus cognitive-behavioral therapy seemed to work better than either approach alone."[4]

In a conversation with me, Jerilyn talked about this turnaround. "We took our staunchest, strictest biological type and put him against our strictest psychological researcher, and we staged a debate," she explained. "And all of a sudden, the psychological person began saying, 'We can't ignore the fact that many of our patients, when they take certain medications, begin doing better in treatment and are getting better.' And then the biological person said, 'Well, medication alone doesn't really cure the disorder, it regulates it. Patients need cognitive-behavioral therapy as well, because if you take the medications away, the symptoms may come back.'

"A lot of the antidepressants, like Prozac, Paxil, and Zoloft, are very useful," Jerilyn continued. "All of these drugs work on the serotonin system. We also know that anti-anxiety medications like Xanax also work. And we have lots of validated studies to show that psychosocial treatments like cognitive-behavioral therapy are effective. But science is still not yet advanced enough to know which treatments work best for which people. Often, treatment proceeds by trial and error. It's important for people to remember that if something doesn't work, it's not that they're a treatment failure. We just haven't found the right combination for them yet.

"You can have two people with the same symptoms and one will do great on Prozac and one will do better on Paxil," she continued. "One will need cognitive-behavioral therapy and one can't do it. The treatment has to be individualized, but these disorders are treatable. Today, we can treat up to 90 percent of people with panic disorder."

When Jerilyn talks about cognitive-behavioral treatment, she is referring to a specific kind of psychotherapy. She writes, "The pioneers in cognitive-behavioral therapy have shown that leading their patients by the hand through situations that induce the most anxious feelings can actually change the chemistry of the brain in powerful, long-lasting, curative ways."[5]

Jerilyn herself was cured using this method. Her therapist, Joe, accompanied her to a high-rise building, the very situation that induced her greatest fears, and together they rode the elevator to the tenth floor, where she remained for fifteen minutes. Joe taught Jerilyn how to deal with her anxiety at the moment she was experiencing it.

In each subsequent session, they would "up the ante" and set a higher floor as a goal. "When my anxiety predictably began to soar," Jerilyn writes about her recovery, "Joe assured me that by staying in the situation and refocusing my thinking, the feelings would pass. He was right.

"Each time this happened, it increased my confidence that, indeed, nothing would happen to me. As frightening as the feelings are, Joe kept reminding me, they are not dangerous."

Jerilyn tried a number of techniques to distract herself from her anxiety and refocus her thoughts. "I can still recall standing on the fifteenth or eighteenth floor of some building, eating sunflower seeds, snapping a rubber band, and frantically counting backward by threes while waiting for the panicky feelings to subside—and hoping against hope that no one would step off the elevator or out of an office and see me!

"But I was on the fifteenth or eighteenth floor, and that was the more important motivating force."[6] Eventually, as I explained in chapter 2, she made it to the top of the Gulf + Western Building in Manhattan.

Today, Jerilyn advocates a form of cognitive therapy that takes a six-point approach:

1. Expect, allow, and accept that fear will rise.
2. When fear comes up, stop, wait, and let it be.
3. Focus on and do manageable things in the present.
4. Label your level of fear from 0 to 10. Watch it go up and down.
5. Function with fear. Appreciate your achievement.
6. Expect, allow, and accept that fear will reappear.

Jerilyn has found this step-by-step procedure, sometimes in combination with the new medical therapies, helpful with countless patients. Statistics from the NIMH suggest that only 23 percent of people with anxiety disorders seek treatment. Yet, according to Jerilyn, using the therapies currently available, "the vast majority of those suffering from these common maladies can be made well enough to function effectively and even joyously."[7]

Obsessive-Compulsive Disorder (OCD)

Until recently, individuals suffering from OCD had little hope for relief from obsessive thoughts (say, that germs are infecting them) and the crippling rituals (repeated hand-washing) that result. The good news is that now there is help for many who suffer.

Researchers have discovered that some antidepressant medications such as Prozac have produced considerable improvements in many people with OCD. Since these medications are the ones that increase the levels of serotonin in the brain, scientists are looking closely at the role this neurotransmitter plays.[8] They have also found that these medications reduce the levels of other brain chemicals that are significantly higher in individuals with OCD and that produce compulsive behaviors in laboratory animals.[9]

The dopamine system might also be involved. A part of the brain that we use in thinking about and planning movement[10] has high concentrations of this neurotransmitter, and if it is damaged, OCD-like symptoms can result.[11]

Research to unlock the secrets of this illness is proceeding on several fronts. Using PET scans, scientists have mapped four areas of the brain that seem to be involved.[12] These are areas that move our thoughts along, tell us when things are right or wrong, and connect with our autonomic (involuntary) responses.

Dr. Jeffrey Schwartz, in his book *Brain Lock,* theorizes that because of genetic or other factors in OCD patients, some of these areas get "stuck in the 'on' position," producing a constant state of over-arousal. When this occurs, the person affected has terrible thoughts and feelings that "something is wrong," which, Dr. Schwartz explains, "lead to compulsive behaviors done in a desperate attempt to make the feelings go away."[13]

Another interesting area of inquiry is that of the influence of a strep throat infection on the development of OCD in children. I was fascinated to learn about this—and about how scientists happen upon and pursue leads in their research.

Dr. Susan Swedo, the acting scientific director of the National Institute of Mental Health, has been studying a small group of children who suddenly developed OCD after infections with a strain of streptococcus. Their disorder is the type that has a "sawtooth" course—it gets better and then worse without a discernible reason (usually OCD symptoms wax and wane with stress).

"I have to credit a patient's mother for this discovery," Dr. Swedo explained during my recent visit to NIMH. "She came to me with a child who had an abrupt explosion of OCD symptoms. Out of the blue he developed strange movements, like flapping his hands. He also started hoarding paper and saliva, and he washed his hands compulsively.

"At first his doctor thought he was doing this for attention," Dr. Swedo said, "but his mother was a medical technologist. She had already decided that her older son's Tourette's syndrome worsened following a strep infection. She came here, and we investigated further."

Dr. Swedo and her research team discovered that infections such as strep throat may trigger an autoimmune response in children who are genetically vulnerable that causes or worsens these sudden cases of childhood OCD. The antibodies that would normally fight the infection instead somehow wrongly attack part of the brain (the basal ganglia), causing inflammation there. Treatments such as cleaning the blood of these antibodies and the administration of medication, even penicillin, can decrease these symptoms.

Dr. Swedo showed me a video of a child with strep-triggered symptoms stumbling about, waving his hands wildly. He was jerking so that he couldn't steady himself enough to walk without help. She then showed me a video of the afflicted boy after treatment. It was amazing. He walked normally with his hands at his sides. After two to four weeks of treatment, the symptoms had been reduced by 60 percent. "We have treated seven kids here who developed OCD after a strep infection, and the immediate treatment effect is profound. After one year, two youngsters are off their medications altogether."

Treatments for Obsessive-Compulsive Disorder

Psychiatrist Jeffrey Schwartz sits at a desk piled high with computer printouts, PET scans, and research papers in a cramped office at UCLA's Neuropsychiatric Institute, talking passionately about his favorite subjects: cognitive-behavioral therapy for obsessive-compulsive disorder, free will, and brain function.

"People with OCD have intrusive thoughts because of a biological, often genetically based brain problem. But how they respond to the false brain messages changes the future messages the brain sends them. If they give in to their obsessions and compulsions, the brain gets worse; if they don't give in, the brain gets better.

"Treatment is not just about finding the right medications. It's a heroic struggle. Look at Winston Churchill. He had manic-depression, but failure was not an option for him. Motivation has a tremendous bearing on the prognosis of a case. Do you give in to your pain, or do you grit your teeth and go through it?

"One of my patients was to appear on a television program with me," he went on. "The show was following her progress for ten weeks. She would leave group therapy sessions saying, 'I've got to do my homework now.' She changed her biology in ten weeks because she was motivated to get well.

"If you change your behavior, you can change your brain chemistry. You can even change the way your DNA expresses itself. Faith has the potential to affect biology; there are things people can do to help themselves, including going to church. There they can find the spiritual wherewithal to overcome their illness. When they change their behavior, they initiate new brain circuits. And the instant a new circuit is activated with treatment, it is a sign of a person's will acting on the brain."

Dr. Schwartz backs up some of his surprising assertions with PET scans taken of patients before and after participating in cognitive-behavioral therapy groups. Even without medication, the "hot spots" in the brain that are overly active when one is in the grips of OCD[14] returned to near normal with therapy. In his book *Brain Lock,* he writes, "For the first time ever for any psychiatric condition or any psychotherapeutic technique, we have scientific evidence that cognitive-behavioral therapy alone actually causes chemical changes in the brains of people with OCD."[15]

Dr. Schwartz's work is noteworthy because he is the first person to actually quantify the effectiveness of psychotherapy using brain scans. Moreover, he has shown that some nonmedical interventions such as cognitive-behavioral therapy can be just as effective in treating OCD as medical interventions.

SSRI medications such as Prozac and Luvox, which enhance the levels of serotonin in the brain, are also helpful in the treatment of OCD. Other useful medications include BuSpar, an anti-anxiety treatment, and clomipramine, an older antidepressant. It may take up to three months, however, for the medications to reach their full effectiveness.

Medication and psychotherapy are complementary, not competitive. We cannot yet predict who will respond to what treatment, but with trial and error, many are helped.

Children with OCD also respond to treatment with Prozac, Luvox, and clomipramine. And, according to Dr. Susan Swedo, those whose illness developed as a result of a strep infection can be effectively treated with immunological treatments such as plasmapheresis (filtering the blood).

❧

Scientists continue to make great progress in the recognition and treatment of anxiety disorders. The most important thing for people suffering from these disorders to know is that they have a serious but treatable problem. They need to know, too, that they are not alone, that their condition is not trivial, and that, with appropriate care, they can expect to lead normal, productive lives.

Part III

Interventions: Preventive, Personal, and Public

*W*ebster's *New World Dictionary* defines intervention as "the act of intervening—coming between as in order to modify, settle or hinder some action." Certainly, we would like to intervene to control mental illnesses, to modify the toll they take on individuals and their families, and eventually to hinder or prevent them.

Today there are exciting possibilities for these interventions. The growth in knowledge about mental illnesses in recent years has significantly increased our understanding of how and why they occur. This, as we have seen, has led to new treatments that better control the illnesses and lessen their severity. It has also allowed us to determine more fully the risks that contribute to their development, and although scientists are not yet in a position to specify definitive strategies, there is enough information to point out some opportunities for preventive intervention.

At our tenth annual mental health symposium at The Carter Center, "Children and Families at Risk," we focused on risk factors that contribute to the onset of mental illness and interventions that reduce these factors and promote mental health, particularly in children.

Dr. William Beardslee, acting chairman of the Department of Psychiatry at Children's Hospital of Boston and professor of child psychiatry at Harvard Medical School, reminded us that historically, a focus on prevention has been neglected, although a good deal of work has been done in the past ten years. From a scientific point of view, the study of prevention involves following, over extended periods, large samples of individuals who are at risk of developing mental disorders. Prevention involves considering what will happen, for instance, three, five, ten, and fifteen years or more down the line. It does not focus on short-term outcomes or what is demonstrable in a single year.

Our society has a difficult time thinking about the future over the long term and in making commitments to follow through with programs. This has contributed to the lack of serious efforts designed to prevent long-term mental health problems.

The Institute of Medicine of the National Academy of Sciences recently examined a series of risk factors for major disorders, including depression. In depression, for instance, the risks range from having a relative who had the disorder (suggesting some kind of genetic cause) to being subjected to severe stress—a loss, divorce, separation, unemployment, or some other traumatic experience. Fifteen years ago, we did not understand the powerful effects that violence and living in poverty have on later mental disorders, including depression. Now we have some sense of these.

As Dr. Beardslee points out, "In trying to understand a . . . disorder's cause and prevention, we are immersed in a sea of social factors (i.e., loss, poverty, unemployment). . . .

"What kinds of evidence, what kinds of conclusions, can we reach about prevention programs for children and adolescents? . . . Whatever preserves the unborn child's biological integrity and psychosocial maturity from conception onward will substantially contribute to the reduction of mental illness later on. Thus, programs such as good prenatal care and immunizations are tremendously important. So are adequate neurological and physical development, a caring relationship with a family member, and some stimulating experiences."

While there is still much to be learned about reducing risks for mental illnesses, there are interventions that have demonstrated effectiveness, as we will see in the following chapter. When we become aware of these interventions, we can apply them in our own families to lessen the risks of family members developing the illnesses.

There are also actions or interventions of a personal nature that families can take to make life easier when one of their members has a serious mental illness. This is particularly important for caregivers, who often neglect their own needs in order to care for a loved one. Caregiving for those who have been thrust into the role can be an extremely lonely, stressful, and frustrating responsibility. They must take care of themselves and have some life outside the caregiving role in order to stay healthy and able, both physically and emotionally, to care for the one who is ill. There are many people in our communities who suffer because of and along with a seriously mentally ill family member who are willing to share advice and help others in similar situations.

Today, these same family members are joining together to publicly advocate better care for those who are mentally ill. They are playing valuable roles in overcoming stigma by educating friends, relatives, and colleagues about mental illnesses and speaking out openly about the issues, and they are seeking out elected officials and letting them know of the needs of their loved ones.

We can all intervene by joining together with family and advocacy groups in our communities to educate people about the true facts of mental illnesses. Our message is that mental illnesses can be diagnosed; they can be treated; and almost all who are affected can lead productive lives. We can also join together to advocate equity in mental health services and insurance—working toward the day when those who suffer will no longer have to face the discrimination that has always been a part of their lives.

Taken together, these interventions—preventive, personal, and public—can make and are making a difference. Mental health has been brought into the mainstream of the public debate on health policy. Today there is much help and much hope for those with mental illnesses and for their families.

Chapter 10

Can We Prevent Mental Illness?

W e know that adequate sewer systems, safe drinking water, and good nutrition all combine to improve dramatically the quality of human life and health. These "protective" measures have reduced illness and death, yet none of them were directed at a specific illness.[1]

We can prevent many things now even though we don't have the complete scientific knowledge about how to treat them. Consider AIDS or fetal alcohol syndrome. We have not yet found cures for these disorders, but we certainly have a clear idea of how they can be prevented.

The question of whether there is anything we can do to prevent mental illness has been one of the most personally pressing for me in the twenty-five years I have spent as a mental health advocate. Having witnessed the human potential wasted by these illnesses, I can't help but be drawn to the issue.

While we must continue to be concerned about sufficient funds for treating mental illnesses, particularly for those who are severely and persistently mentally ill, developing ways to reduce their prevalence and perhaps even prevent some of them is a goal that must be pursued.

The research of the last decade or so has taught us much about the brain and, as we learned earlier, has enabled us to develop far more effective medications than we have had in the past. We should continue to encourage research, not only to improve treatment, but also with the idea that it may enable us to develop preventive interventions.

It has been historically difficult to generate support for the prevention of mental illness and promotion of mental health. I have been encouraged, however, by signs of increasing attention. The publication in 1994 of *Reducing Risks for Mental Disorders: Frontiers for Preventive Intervention Research,* a report prepared under the auspices of the Institute of Medicine of the National Academy of Sciences, represents one of the most thorough reviews of the field of prevention with regard to mental disorders. The report makes clear that we are indeed making progress in the field, but points out that there is much more we need to learn.

What Is Prevention?

In 1978, the President's Commission on Mental Health looked at the issue of prevention from a social point of view—how people's lives are affected by their environment. We discussed the effects of poverty and malnutrition, of living in the slums of cities surrounded by drugs and crime; of broken homes due to death or divorce; of living in homes where parents are alcoholics or drug addicts, where they quarrel too much and where there is little love; of being unemployed; of poor schools and discrimination of all types.

Today, because of our remarkable new knowledge about the brain, there are exciting possibilities for prevention, and efforts are being concentrated not just on one's life circumstances, but also on research to identify and reduce biological risk factors for specific disorders.

Already, with the significant progress that has been made in medications and treatments, the symptoms of mental illnesses—even the major illnesses—have been dramatically reduced. Much of the recurrence and the debilitating effects of mental illnesses can now be prevented. The side effects of medication are lessened, and so many who in the past were doomed to a lifetime of illness are now able to live productive lives. There is also no doubt that being able to control mental illnesses prevents many of the most serious consequences, even suicide.

The ultimate goal of research, of course, is to understand enough about the disorders to prevent them from occurring in the first place.[2] Scientists have been studying, for example, the effects of childhood stress on the adult behavior of primates, who are genetically closest to humans, and their serotonin systems. They are trying to better understand whether there is a correlation between stress and low levels of serotonin on the one hand and depression, alcoholism, aggression, and suicide on the other.[3]

As a result of studies with humans, researchers are learning more about the important interconnections among school achievement, conduct disorders, and depression in small children and adolescents.[4]

Other scientists are exploring the theory that different neurotransmitters are activated at different stages of development. Serotonin systems, for example, mature early, while the dopamine system implicated in schizophrenia seems to develop much more gradually and only reaches maturity at adolescence. This may explain why schizophrenia symptoms usually become manifest at this time of life.[5]

Immunization may become a significant strategy in the future to prevent mental illness. According to Richard Jed Wyatt, chief of the neuropsychiatry branch at NIMH, more than a dozen research studies have linked a mother's infection with influenza during the second trimester of pregnancy with the subsequent development of schizophrenia. "If more evidence supporting this association becomes available, widespread immunization of women of childbearing age against influenza could become an important act of prevention for schizophrenia," he writes.[6] And Dr. Susan Swedo's exciting new work with obsessive-compulsive disorder and strep infections at NIMH might also give rise to an anti-OCD vaccine for children in the future.

Immunization would represent primary prevention in its traditional sense—that is, an activity that attempts to eliminate the cause of a mental disorder. Today primary prevention encompasses a broad range of actions that either ward off a disorder or foster good health in order to decrease the development of new cases.

The spectrum of preventive interventions includes:

• *Universal.* These preventive measures are desirable for everyone in the general public and for all members of a specific group, such as pregnant women, the elderly, or children. Usually these measures can be applied without professional advice. They might include good nutrition, prenatal care, Head Start programs, assertiveness training, and substance abuse programs.

• *Selective.* These preventive measures apply to individuals in subgroups of the population who might be at particular risk. Age, gender, occupation, family history, or life situation would identify these subgroups. Pregnant teenagers (and their soon-to-be-born children), for example, might benefit from selective intervention programs.

• *Indicated.* These preventive measures are directed at individuals who, although they do not yet experience symptoms, have a lifestyle, condition, or abnormality that identifies them as being at high risk for the future development of a mental disorder. A program for youngsters who fail in school, exhibit early behavior problems, and are alienated from their families would be an indicated intervention.

The Role of Risk Factors

The 1994 Institute of Medicine (IOM) study on the prevention of mental illnesses was done at the request of Congress. The institute reviewed all the work in the field and reported their recommendations in order to coordinate research and delivery of services into the twenty-first century. The IOM's Committee on the Prevention of Mental Disorders surveyed developments in neuroscience, genetics, epidemiology, and child development.

They came to the conclusion that currently there is little evidence from research that any *specific* mental disorder can be prevented. However, they added that there is "considerable evidence that certain risk factors of mental disorders have been clearly identified."[7]

Risk factors are characteristics or hazards that, if present, may make it more likely for an individual to develop a mental disorder. For example, being fired from a job would be a risk factor for depression and substance abuse. Factors that may place someone at risk at one stage in life may not be as harmful at another.[8] Compare, for instance, the emotional impact that the death of a mother might have on an infant's well-being in contrast to the loss of one's mother when well into middle age. Or consider the impact of a teenager fired from a summer job because of being late compared to the effect on a fifty-seven-year-old plant manager of being laid off due to downsizing.

As the IOM report points out, scientists have identified factors that put one at risk for many, but not all, mental disorders and related problems (substance abuse and violence). They have also identified many factors that may protect us.

Altering Risk Factors

To understand how we might be able to positively influence some risk factors, consider the *illness prevention/health promotion* approach to physical illness that we know so well: to avoid heart disease, we are all aware that we should reduce fat and cholesterol in our diets and eat more fresh fruits, vegetables, and whole grains; exercise; maintain an ideal weight; and stop smoking. If these measures fail, we may take cholesterol-lowering medications. Although we may have a genetic predisposition to cardiovascular disease, by our behaviors we can reduce the risks while we strengthen the factors that may protect us from a heart attack.

All of the preventive measures that we take to help preserve our physical health are based on years of public health research—research that has not been carried out to the same degree in the field of mental health.

Yet despite the fact that prevention research in the mental health field is still a very new area of scientific investigation, we need to be aware of the risk factors and protective factors that have already been identified. And we need to apply this knowledge where we can.

What Are the Risk Factors?

In part II, we explored the brain's "plasticity"—its amazing capacity to change in response to its environment, both for good and bad. Experiences and learning, medications, substance abuse, and probably prenatal "events" and infectious diseases may all play a role in altering brain circuits. Nerve cells may strengthen, grow new connections, or shrink depending on what one learns or remembers. The way we interact with our children may even have a profound effect. Recently I watched a video showing differences in toddlers' brains depending upon whether their mothers screamed at them for touching a valuable object or calmly corrected the behavior and redirected the child's attention. The contrast in brain wiring was surprising—a good example of how nature and nurture interact to shape the brain.

According to the National Institutes of Health, risk factors for mental illnesses, therefore, may "reside within the individual or within the family, social network, community or institutions that surround the individual." They may be biological and/or psychosocial (related to one's social environment).[9]

Biological risk factors may include:

- *Genetics.* One's inheritance may increase vulnerability to mental illnesses.
- *Prenatal "insults."* A mother's struggle with influenza or severe malnutrition may cause abnormalities in the development of her baby's brain during gestation. Rh incompatibility may also be a factor.
- *Extremely low birth weight.*
- *Biological "insults."* There are sensitive periods during children's development when they are particularly vulnerable to sensory and emotional deprivation, physical trauma, malnutrition, and exposure to toxic chemicals or drugs.
- *Chronic physical illnesses.* Leukemia, diabetes, asthma, cystic fibrosis, epilepsy, and AIDS have been linked to a vulnerability to mental illnesses, as have chronic physical conditions such as blindness and deafness.[10]

We know that risk factors are not biological alone. If they were, when one of a pair of identical twins becomes ill with schizophrenia, the other one would invariably become ill, too. Instead, approximately 50 percent of the others actually develop the disorder.[11]

Psychosocial risk factors include:

- Poor prenatal care, which can increase the risk of prematurity and low birth weight
- Extreme poverty, which can increase the risk of prematurity, malnutrition, inadequate health care and housing, and lack of parental support
- Very young or immature mothers who lack well-developed parenting skills
- Low intelligence and learning disabilities
- Persistent social adversity, low social status, disorganized and inadequate schooling, homelessness, violence, and over-crowded living conditions
- Traumatic events such as assault, rape, domestic violence, catastrophic accidents, natural disasters, or wartime experiences, which can all lead to post-traumatic stress disorder (severe anxiety, nightmares, flashbacks, depression)
- Child abuse or neglect, which has been correlated with depression, the inability to form healthy attachments, the failure to develop a healthy conscience, and violent behavior in adulthood
- A child placed in foster care or moved from one foster care situation to another is at risk for "reactive attachment disorder" (difficulty in building bonds with others), a condition psychologists say comes from a purely environmental influence: the absence of a nurturing caregiver in the earliest, most vulnerable stage of life[12]

- Disturbed family relationships including severe marital discord, parental criminality, and domestic violence, which are emotionally scarring and may lead to conduct disorder in children and antisocial personality disorder in adults (a pattern of irresponsible, impulsive, violent, and remorseless behavior)
- Parental mental illness, which may lead to traumatic disruptions in family life and inconsistent parenting. Studies have also shown that infants born to depressed mothers have elevated stress hormones, brain activity suggestive of depression, and depressive symptoms such as loss of appetite and disturbed sleep[13]

Although biological risk factors may be somewhat more fixed, many of the psychological and social risk factors may be responsive to change. It is important to bear in mind, however, that what happens at one stage of a child's development doesn't necessarily dictate a poor outcome at a later stage. *Having risk factors in one's life does not guarantee that one will develop a mental illness.* This is one of the most significant and hopeful of the IOM's findings.[14] Risk does not mean destiny.

Nevertheless, once people become aware of the dangers, they may be able to take action to address the situation. For example:

- Pregnant women need to be encouraged to visit the doctor for regular pre- and post-natal visits.
- Parents should do all they can to encourage their teenagers to abstain from sexual activity or to protect themselves from unwanted pregnancy.
- New mothers and their babies should be given as much emotional support as possible.

• Parents who suspect their child has a learning disability should be persistent about pursuing early diagnosis and treatment. Untreated disabilities can create a lifetime of low self-esteem, depression, and even incarceration.

• Anyone who has experienced a traumatic event such as the ones listed above should seek counseling as soon as possible. Post-traumatic stress disorder can be helped with prompt treatment.

• Anyone who recognizes child abuse (physical, sexual, or emotional), domestic violence, or severe marital discord in the family should seek therapy, education, and/or other interventions.

• Individuals with family histories of a particular mental illness should be vigilant for early warning signs that signal the development of a problem. Early intervention in mental illness can help ensure a more positive prognosis.

• Drug and alcohol abuse may be indications that someone is suffering from a mental disorder.

Protective Factors

Even when risk factors can't be changed, the good news is that we might be able to strengthen protective factors to lessen our chances of becoming ill.[15] We all need to learn to nurture our family's mental health as carefully as our physical health. Just as there are critical periods of sensitivity to risk factors, so are there critical periods for protective factors, especially for children.

In February 1996, we brought together scores of mental health advocates and professionals at The Carter Center to discuss how we could develop a strategy for a national movement committed to improving children's lives.[16] We developed a consensus on what communities need to help children achieve a high level of success:

- Economic and physical security, within the home and neighborhood
- Environmental and public safety
- A nurturing, stable family environment
- Adult mentors and role models in the community
- Positive peer activities
- The opportunity to exert effort and achieve success
- Health care for medical needs
- Decent schools and schooling
- Access to services to treat needs that may arise and require professional care[17]

This does not mean that all children raised in nurturing communities where strong protective factors are present will escape mental disorders, nor does it mean that all children raised in communities without such protective factors will have poor outcomes. It does mean, however, that the absence of any of these conditions puts children at greater risk—the fewer the protective factors, the greater the risk.

But more than just the absence of abuse, neglect, or other environmental dangers, all children need opportunities to experience growth and receive reinforcement to do well—they need loving care and support as they grow.

Why Focus on Children?

When we talk about the prevention of mental illnesses, we most often talk about children. The reason is quite logical. It is far easier to intervene early than it is to deal with the consequences of poverty, neglect, violence, and abuse after they have taken their toll.[18]

Early interventions aimed at all children increase the likelihood that when life's stresses and other negative environmental influences occur, they will not have as potent an effect.[19] A child's early years are crucial for the promotion of mental health.

• Children's brain development before the age of one is rapid and extensive. Although the cells have formed before birth, they continue to mature long after birth.

• Children's brain development is much more vulnerable to environmental influence than that of adults. Malnutrition and other "insults," such as exposure to lead poisoning, before birth and during the first year of life can lead to neurological and behavioral disorders.

• Environment also affects the number of brain cells and connections as well as how these are "wired."

• A child's early environment can have lifelong consequences. Infants exposed to good nutrition, appropriate toys, and playmates have measurably better brain function at the age of twelve than those who were not.

• Early stress can permanently affect brain function, memory, and learning. Children who experience extreme stress early in their lives are at greater risk for mental, behavioral, and emotional difficulties later in life.[20]

Effective intervention with children can delay the onset of a mental illness. This is important, because research has shown that about half of those who have had a single depressive episode will go on to have more.[21] The longer one can delay the appearance of the first episode, the better. Early intervention may also break a cycle of abuse, neglect, violence, drug use, and poverty for future generations. The old adage "An ounce of prevention is worth a pound of cure" still applies.

Children need protection and nurturing. As parents you can provide your own early interventions, such as creating a loving and respect-filled home and stressing the importance of a healthy mind and body. You can open the lines of communication so that your children come to you with their problems and fears. You can watch for the signs of substance abuse and seek out mental health services promptly (and without shame) if you fear that something is amiss. An unhappy five-year-old, if not helped, may in time grow into a self-destructive fifteen-year-old.

Adolescence, in particular, is a time to be wary. This is when many mental illnesses first emerge, so you will want to pay close attention to sources of stress. Be alert if your teenager exhibits any of the following behaviors:

- Trouble in maintaining social connections or a sudden change in peer groups
- Refusal to participate in family activities
- Poor school performance, including cutting classes or losing interest in favorite subjects
- Persistent anger, restlessness, irritability, aggressiveness, or loss of interest in physical appearance
- Extreme sensitivity about eating or food
- Changes in appetite and sleep habits
- Intense reactions to rejection or loss
- Extreme anxiety
- Drug or alcohol abuse
- Involvement with gangs, violence, or stealing

Of course, many of these behaviors are typical teen responses to hormonal changes, changing social roles, and the move away from parents toward greater independence. How do you know if your child is out of the norm? Follow your instincts. If you feel that something is wrong, talk to the school counselor or a qualified therapist to get more information. Take your child for an evaluation if you're not sure. Remember, depression is often overlooked in teens because it is written off as typical teen anger. It is better to err on the side of caution than wait too long to get help.

Early Intervention in the Community

The most important advances in early intervention must come from our communities, and this will only happen when we develop the political will to bring small, model community-based programs to scale and make children our first priority.

At our tenth annual mental health symposium at The Carter Center, in November 1994, we convened leaders from the fields of education, business, health, juvenile justice, and the faith communities to discuss children and families at risk. We focused on what can be done in our local communities to reduce the problems confronting children and their families, especially violence, substance abuse, mental and emotional disorders, and those factors that impede a child's readiness to learn.

Dr. William Beardslee, professor of child psychiatry at Harvard Medical School, was a member of the IOM Committee on Prevention. He told us that "to wait until children become ill is to wait far too long."[22] Even the World Bank has become supportive of early intervention. This international body has found that integrated programs—those that strive to address all of a child's basic needs, including food, clothing, and shelter as well as health care, affection, intellectual stimulation, and opportunities that promote learning—can do much to prevent stunted cognitive development and insufficient preparation for school. "Thirty years of research have shown that such programs can improve primary and even secondary school performance, increase children's prospects for higher productivity and future income, and reduce the probability that they will become burdens on public health and social service budgets."[23]

Early intervention in the community can mean:

- Improving a pregnant mother's diet and helping her stop smoking or engaging in other damaging activities
- Helping mothers of premature infants to stimulate their babies appropriately
- Teaching parents, especially those who have been abused themselves, how to improve interactions with their children and how to respond to youngsters' needs
- Providing job programs for parents and other initiatives to raise parents' self-esteem
- Showing parents how to help their children achieve in school
- Teaching children coping and decision-making skills—especially when facing peer pressure

Early community intervention also means that we must all work together. At our conference, Dr. Beardslee emphasized that "building alliances across agencies, groups, families, schools, individuals, hospitals, and community institutions is the best way to develop prevention strategies. Prevention intervention should focus on the community in planning and implementation.

"People do not exist in isolation," he said. "We will move forward only insofar as we are able to work together."

Community Prevention Programs That Work

At our symposium on children and families at risk, we heard many frightening statistics about the increase in poverty and violence, and the resulting potential for mental illness among children and families within our communities. But the panelists also made it clear that we now know much more about strategies for intervention, and that early intervention is a key starting point.

We also heard uplifting stories of programs that work, where people have joined together in their communities to make good things happen. At the core of each one of these programs is an effort to enhance the self-esteem of children at risk and help their parents and community members develop specific problem-solving skills and competencies.

Dr. Beardslee told us about some of the programs the Institute of Medicine studied for its report. One in Baltimore, run by Dr. Shep Kellum, has used special mentoring sessions, extra classroom time and attention, and similar interventions in the public school to help children overcome learning deficits. Dr. Kellum has shown that when a child's reading ability increases, that child's likelihood of developing depressive symptoms decreases. Another program, which was also linked to the schools, is in Tacoma, Washington. Called Homebuilders, it seeks to keep together families who are at risk of disintegration. Families at risk not served by the program were three times more likely to have youngsters placed outside the home as those in the program.[24] Linking families and schools seems tremendously important.

Mark Rosenberg, director of the National Center for Injury Prevention and Control at the Centers for Disease Control, told us that when nurses go into homes and instruct new parents on child care and parenting techniques, they can make a real difference in preventing child abuse and reducing the chances of subsequent violent behavior. He also reminded us that programs for preschoolers like Head Start and others that teach social skills in combination with mentoring can increase children's ability to engage in nonviolent conflict resolution and decrease their aggressive behavior.[25]

Dr. Joycelyn Elders, the former Surgeon General of the United States, shared with us the story of a "wellness clinic" at Central High School in Little Rock, Arkansas. "Forty percent of the services offered in this school-based health clinic are related to mental health," she explained. They have thirteen different counseling groups—dealing with issues from stress management and drug and alcohol abuse to male responsibility.

"One young man," she related, "told me, 'They are teaching us that we need to respect girls and open the door for them, and that we need to treat them nice. I did not know we were supposed to do all that.' Another said, 'This wellness clinic is like having parents in school.' What could be better than feeling you have parents and loving guidance at school with you all day?"[26]

I am personally familiar with one of the most interesting programs described that day. It is in a high school in a gang-infested neighborhood in the Washington Heights section of Manhattan, where it is not safe to walk from your car to the school. Madeleine Kunin, deputy secretary of the U.S. Department of Education, described it. "The minute you are in the school," she said, "you are in a cheerful, safe, disciplined, happy place where learning is going on at full speed. The school is open until 10:30 P.M. and welcomes students as well as their parents, 90 percent of whom are from the Dominican Republic. Parents take English lessons and learn about computers. And the New York City Children's Aid Society has established medical and dental clinics on campus."[27]

I visited this school one day to view their immunization and health programs for preschool children. It was a happy place. In the clinic, well babies were getting their checkups and immunizations and sick babies were getting care. I met with young mothers attending parenting classes and with grandmothers being taught about nutrition as they learned English. I left thinking what a difference it would make if all our schools could be like this one!

Another program, called AVANCE, which serves five thousand families in poverty in San Antonio, Texas, had its beginning because of one young woman's frustration with the school system. Gloria Rodriguez was a teacher who saw too many young people dropping out of school and too much violence and substance abuse. Gloria decided to try to do something about it. She created AVANCE. "We begin with parents who have children under the age of three," she said. "We help them learn all they can about child growth and development. They make educational toys, books, puppets, balls, playhouses, hobby-horses, all with the purpose of teaching concepts and skills that will get children ready for school. We have bilingual curriculum in all areas of development."

The parents are taught principles of child development, from the importance of love to the health needs of children. They learn how to play with their youngsters and how to get them ready for school. The program also connects these families with over a hundred different service agencies. Their research has revealed that those involved in the program are more nurturing and more responsive to their children. "More than forty percent of the children from these high-crime, high-risk areas are growing up and going on to college," Dr. Rodriguez explained.

She told us about one mother who said to her, "I don't know what life would be like if I had not come to AVANCE. Maybe I would be in a mental institution, maybe I would be on drugs, or maybe I would be a prostitute on Guadalupe Street. [She had been on drugs; she had been a prostitute; before she came to AVANCE her two children were about to be taken from her.] Somehow, AVANCE came into my life and gave me hope and gave me the right kind of support and the person I was then, I am no longer."[28]

All of these programs have in common efforts to reduce the risk factors that can contribute to mental illness while they enhance protective factors that can help keep our children well.

Promotion of Mental Health and Resiliency

Though primary prevention has come to include the prevention of mental illness and the promotion of mental health, they are not identical pursuits, but they do intertwine. Prevention strives to ward off the development of mental illness, whereas promotion seeks to enhance our strengths, abilities, skills, and ultimately our self-esteem. Promotion equips individuals to cope more effectively with life's challenges and adversities, encouraging wellness. It is a positive approach rather than a reaction to deficits. Activities as simple as participation in religious services, physical exercise, and recreation have all been cited as ways to enhance mental well-being.

According to long-time prevention advocate Beverly Long, "the promotion of mental health may prove to be the best preventive measure we can take. For instance, scientific research shows that health promotion through effective socialization in families, classrooms, and peer groups appears not only to benefit all children, but specifically to increase protective factors among vulnerable children. If young people can be taught to deal with emotional stresses before they turn into serious problems, some later mental health problems can be averted."

Recently, research has turned toward trying to understand why some youngsters who grow up in difficult environments reach maturity relatively unscathed. Not only do they not suffer from mental illness, but they also have an unusual capacity to recover from significant stress.[29] These remarkable youngsters have been called "resilient children." They emerge from high-risk situations with their self-esteem intact and are blessed with the capacity to work well, play well, love well, and expect well.

Dr. Beardslee has been studying resilient children who have a depressed parent. "We found," he said, "that youngsters with parents suffering from depression who were resilient had close confiding relationships with others. They were interpersonally connected. They also were activists and doers outside the home. They were not trapped at home, but felt that they could move forward. Furthermore, they had developed a profound understanding of the parent's illness. They believed they were neither the cause of their parent's illness, nor to blame for it. This understanding was crucial to their coping. Generally, they saw themselves as separate—both from the illness and from their affected parent—and were able to act independently."

Dr. John Gates,[30] the director of our mental health program at The Carter Center, is a strong advocate for promoting resilience in children. He explains that resiliency is akin to the concept of wellness. "All people, not just those at risk, stand to profit from wellness enhancement," he says. In fact, the original goals of the Head Start program, some thirty years ago, echo the characteristics that now define resiliency.

Resilient children:

• *Are socially competent.* They are responsive, flexible, empathetic, caring, with good communication skills, a sense of humor, and an ability to elicit positive responses from others.

• *Have problem-solving skills.* They are able to think abstractly and reflectively and develop alternate solutions to cognitive and social problems.

• *Are autonomous.* Independent, they have a sense of self-esteem and self-discipline and feel that they have the power to exert some influence over their environment.

• *Possess a sense of purpose and a future.* They have healthy expectations, goals, and motivation for career and education achievement. They are persistent and hopeful and have a sense of a compelling future.[31]

They have also been described as having a determined approach to problem-solving; a tendency to evaluate experiences constructively even in the face of adversity; and the ability to view life and their future as meaningful.[32]

These characteristics, combined with stable support from caregivers, seem to protect children, enabling them to cope effectively with adverse circumstances as diverse as poverty, divorce, mental illness, addiction, and war. Dr. Gates tells us that resilient children are in a sense "immunized—they are more resistant to the ill effects of life's stresses and risks."

How can your children acquire such resiliency? It is more likely to occur if your family, their schools, and communities foster healthy development in children and adolescents. In *Today's Children: Creating a Future for a Generation in Crisis,* Dr. David Hamburg lists seven factors that may contribute to resiliency, although we recognize that they may not be attainable for all children:

1. An intact, cohesive family that can be depended upon in every crunch

2. Multifaceted parent–child relationships with at least one parent who is consistently nurturing and loving and able to enjoy child-rearing, teaching, and coping

3. Supportive extended family members who are available to lend a hand

4. A supportive community, whether it be a neighborhood or religious, ethnic, or political group

5. Parents' previous experience with child-rearing during their own years of growth and development for what amounts to an ongoing education for parenthood

6. A child's ability to perceive future opportunities and a tangible basis for envisioning an attractive future

7. A reasonably predictable adult environment that fosters gradual preparation for adult life[33]

High expectations for achievement coupled with caring support from parents and teachers may also create a positive environment.

❧

Today, we may not know how to prevent mental illnesses, but scientists are making great strides toward that goal. In the meantime, while acknowledging that there is still much to be learned about reducing the risks for violence, substance abuse, and mental disorders, there are interventions, especially early childhood interventions, that have demonstrated their effectiveness. While we cannot fully quantify in dollars and cents the savings produced by early intervention, research has consistently shown that preventing problems is much easier than treating them once they are entrenched. The creative programs such as those just described illustrate the possibilities and give us a strong sense of hope that we can develop resilient children, who will in turn grow into resilient adults.

As Dr. Julius Richmond,[34] one of our country's great leaders in every area of child care, has said, "If we figure out ways to replicate our successes, to repeat our joys, to promote our best efforts, we can make a difference in the lives of children. . . . In our national interest, in our personal interest, it is time to apply what we know."

Chapter 11

Caregiving for Mental Illness

Reverend John Rex, minister of the Unitarian Universalist Fellowship in Fredricksburg, Virginia, wrote of the toll mental illness took on his twenty-five-year-old-son, Chris, who had manic-depressive illness that, sadly, did not respond to lithium. "When a family member is suffering, the whole family suffers. . . . We lived those years day-by-day, against increasing mental illness that ran its course, never letting up."

Reverend Rex sent me a copy of a sermon he delivered a year after Chris's death in 1995 of undetermined causes, in which he quoted from a report he had written for the medical inquiry:

> In the summer of 1991 . . . Chris went to a Buffalo Bills game from which he walked home. . . . over twenty miles, in his bare feet in the middle of the night. The next day, while we were calling Crisis Services, he was off wandering, visiting people in the neighborhood. At one house, he jumped in the swimming pool with his clothes on and then called to tell me he would go to the hospital.
>
> I picked him up and drove him, soaking wet, to Buffalo General, where we waited for hours in the emergency waiting room . . . the eventual evaluation showed

he should be hospitalized, but we were told that there was no bed for him . . . [that we should] take him home and bring him back next morning. Dazed and amazed, I walked out the door with him and asked him to wait by the entrance while I walked to get the car (he was in bare and swollen feet). When I drove [back to get him] . . . I was surprised to see a body lying in the middle of the road. As I got closer, I saw that it was Chris. . . . He got in the car. . . .

When we arrived at home, both my wife and I were very upset, not knowing how we would make it through the night. When we called Crisis Services to ask for advice, they told us that they could not intervene if we were not in danger. Just as we were talking . . . Chris smashed the VCR in the next room and was turning over furniture . . . the woman on the phone called the State Police, and they came promptly. Chris elected to go to the hospital, strapped on a stretcher, in an ambulance, with police guard. . . .

I followed in my car, and found myself in the waiting room with Chris. . . . [We] sat with the crowds of others for at least two hours. . . . As I waited there with him, I knew that there is a Hell. We were there. It is not possible for existence to be more terrible.

Countless others across the nation have endured similar emergencies. Coping with the needs of a loved one who has a severe mental illness can be a daunting task. I know this from working in the mental health field for so many years, and from the studies of caregiving I have been involved in since leaving the White House.

When we came home, I learned that our local state university, Georgia Southwestern, had a small endowment for a mental health program. When I was approached with a proposal to establish the Rosalynn Carter Institute (RCI) on the campus, since I already had a mental health program at The Carter Center, it seemed natural to focus on the caregiving aspect of mental illness, which is so often ignored.

Through our studies and research at RCI, I have seen first-hand how difficult caregiving is and how important it is for caregivers to take care of themselves. Many become so absorbed in caring for an ill loved one that they neglect their own needs. Over a period of time, they often reach a state of utter exhaustion, and the quality of care they are able to give is diminished. After much work at the Institute, I wrote a book called *Helping Yourself Help Others,* to provide support to those giving care and to help ease their pain and sense of isolation, to let them know they are not alone.

In chapter 4, I wrote about what you can do when someone you love has a mental illness. Most of those issues pertain to the loved one and the knowledge and information you will need to be able to guide and manage his or her care. This chapter is about you and your needs. In it, I will share with you information from *Helping Yourself Help Others* and from other sources that might be helpful. I will explore some of the issues that may overwhelm you as a caregiver. Where I can, I will suggest ways of dealing with them—not necessarily to resolve them completely, because some may be impossible to correct fully—in the hope of lessening the burden that you face and helping you gain the courage and strength to be an effective caregiver.

The Impact of Mental Illness on the Family

Living with someone who is mentally ill can be an enormous strain on you and your family—the more severe and intense the symptoms, the greater the burden. Every aspect of your lives can be affected: your emotions, work, leisure, financial status, health, relationships with extended family, friends, and neighbors,[1] and even the sense of control over your own lives.

One desperate woman who wrote to me about her plight was plagued by many of these problems:

> My husband had been a successful businessman. . . . We discovered last June that he has a severe mental disorder. This was discovered when Jack was arrested when he tried to bring illegal drugs into this country. He was dressed in his business suit and had driven his Mercedes virtually into the Rio Grande. It made no sense; Jack was always so law-abiding.
>
> The court appointed a doctor who said Jack's mental problems caused his bizarre behavior. He had been going out of control for a while. I did not know what was wrong with him. Our family doctor could not tell us either. Jack can be normal, now that the Bureau of Prisons finally got his medicine right.
>
> Before this we lived in the best neighborhood. We had a Mercedes and a Bronco, a swimming pool, beautiful furniture, a luxury ski condo, vacations, a good life. Our babies were in private schools. Now my husband is in prison, his business is bankrupt, and the vehicles are gone. I have four little babies at home—three are still in diapers—with no car. Going to the grocery store is almost impossible. . . . I have sold all the nice furniture, have no money, insurance. . . . I am taking antidepressants. I'm worried about myself.
>
> Our four-year-old has been in therapy because of the trauma. The five-year-old is back in diapers.

We would feel better if this story were fiction. Unfortunately, it is not.

You and your family may also experience a wide range of difficult and stressful situations when your loved one's mental illness manifests itself. The person who was always healthy and dependable is now irrational, unable to function, possibly self-destructive, and perhaps even absent—wandering the streets, or incarcerated as Jack was. The illness may interfere with your familiar habits and daily activities and temporarily—or permanently—throw lives into chaos. Your life course may be dictated by the whims of the ill one's disorder. This is truly frightening.

The behaviors associated with severe mental illnesses, such as delusions, hallucinations, manic fervor, impaired judgment, poor handling of money, lapses in grooming, obsessions, even apathy and withdrawal, can be highly disturbing and often embarrassing to you and your family members.[2]

A friend whom I have known for many years recently wrote to me about her experiences as a child when her sister had what was then termed a nervous breakdown. "These events of my early life have had a lasting impact on me," she wrote. "Sometimes, I feel we need to hear from the siblings of those afflicted with mental illness. They are the forgotten ones, and they also are in great need because of this illness in the family."

She began her story by writing, "I sat down in church with the girls my age—girls that should have been my friends. Maybe they thought they were my friends, but to me, I felt ostracized from them. Nothing was right in my world. My constant waking moments were full of self-doubt and shame. . . .

"[A] crisis which my young mind had never heard of before had occurred. One of my sisters, who was eight years older than I, had a psychotic break. Wilma was suddenly uprooted from all reality, and for no apparent reason. Sitting down on that bench at church, with the girls my own age, meant more shame to me, because Wilma was sitting on the next bench, acting strange. Her bizarre and erratic behavior included hearing voices, even during the church services, and she would talk back to them, causing my friends to giggle and look at me. After these many years, I still do not know if they were looking to see how I would react, or whether they thought they would observe the same behavior in me.

"So being in church, a place that should lend a safe haven for the distraught, instead was a place of dread. There was no one there who could encourage, counsel, or support this ten-year-old in any way. In fact, at times my embarrassment was almost beyond me when some adult would ask me how Wilma acted at home. There was nowhere to turn for refuge. . . . I had no reason to believe anyone cared. Our family felt only blame for what had happened to Wilma. . . . [T]hey were so entwined with their own shock and heartbreak that it didn't occur to them that the siblings of the afflicted one also needed care and understanding."

Parents, as I'm sure Wilma's did, often suffer from "chronic sorrow," a never-ending grieving process in which they mourn the lost potential of their ill child. Peggy MacGregor, a clinical social worker in Philadelphia whose son was diagnosed with a mental illness, writes about parental grief at this stage. "Because the loss with mental illness is psychosocial and not physical, the community often does not perceive the family's loss and does not expect or join in with expressions of sadness and pain. There are no social or religious rituals to offer as consolation. In addition, because mental illness is a stigmatized disease, the family's own sense of shame may inhibit their right to grieve in their own eyes . . . and friends may be embarrassed to become involved."[3]

One group of researchers has described schizophrenia as "an ungraspable, deathlike calamity, not only to psychotic patients, but also to their kin."[4] This was especially true before the advent of the new medications. Yet Peggy MacGregor notes that family members who express their pain tend to be seen as "unduly self-absorbed." As a result, they are often left to deal with their sorrow alone.[5]

In addition to the isolation and all of the problems the family is experiencing because of the illness, discord can occur among family members themselves. It can be the result of disagreements over the behavior of the ill one and how to handle specific situations, especially when the illness is severe. Even small disagreements that are normal in all families can be highly magnified when everyone is under such stress.

Through our work at RCI, including a survey we did of caregivers in our area, we have found that often family meetings can help ease these situations. Getting family members together (with or without the ill one) can give everyone a chance to express their feelings honestly and openly and relieve any pent-up tensions. These meetings can also provide a chance to include all members of the family in decisions that have to be made— about things as simple as what time to have dinner or other issues as complex as how to handle and adapt to the habits of the one who is ill—things the family has never had to think about before, such as eating and sleeping habits, and sometimes bizarre behavior. If the family is to stay strong, each member's feelings must be considered and some balance maintained in the relationships. Too much time focused on the ill one, for instance, can cause others to feel ignored.

All will need to accept the fact that everything about their daily lives and relationships has changed and that each one will have to make adjustments to accommodate the changes. Keeping everyone not only informed but a part of the decision-making process seems to be the best way to maintain a semblance of family harmony. It's worth a try.

Caring for someone with a mental illness is not easy; it is a challenging task. You and your family may have a difficult road ahead, but there are many others who travel it with you, and much help and information that can guide you along the way.

The Stages of Caregiving

There are many ways to look at the caregiving experience. Dr. Carolyn L. Lindgren, an associate professor at Wayne State University College of Nursing, has studied the "Caregiver Career," especially among those caring for Alzheimer's patients. I think we can generalize her findings for caregivers of all individuals with mental disorders. Her research looks at the experience in stages[6]:

The Encounter Stage

This is the moment when you first get the news of your family member's diagnosis, and it's a time of high stress for everyone. You may struggle to understand what the disorder will mean to the loved one who is ill, to yourself and your family. You may realize at this point that your life has changed, perhaps forever. And, if the ill one is a spouse, you may come to the difficult realization that the natural give-and-take in the relationship has become unbalanced, at least for the moment.

The Encounter Stage is filled with fear and disruption. You may suddenly have to deal with hospitals, doctors, treatments, and a complex maze of services with which you are unfamiliar—all the issues I have discussed in chapter 4.

Your reaction may be one of shock and disbelief before you can slowly come to terms with reality. Most caregivers also feel enormous sadness and a deep personal loss. And although your life is filled with grief and pain, unfortunately you may not find much support at this stage. Professionals and other family members may be focused on helping the one who is ill, and you may not feel that you can express your needs. What you need most in this stage is information. When you learn about the disease and the issues involved, you may gain a sense of control over the situation.

The Enduring Stage

This next stage is the long-term, hard-work phase of caregiving. You have come to terms with the diagnosis and are now engaged daily in the job of providing care. Depending on your loved one's illness and needs, you may find that the time you used to spend on activities you enjoyed on your own has dwindled. And you are likely to become so engrossed in your caregiving responsibilities that you begin to lose contact with friends and family. It is at this point—especially if your family member is struggling with a major mental illness—that you might feel hopeless and despairing, frustrated and lost. You might give little thought to yourself or to the future.

During the Enduring Stage, however, it's most important for you to set aside time to take care of yourself, especially if the demands of caregiving surpass your inner resources.

The Exit Stage

At this point, the caregiving role diminishes or ends. Hopefully, your ill family member may return to a more normal state. This is the best of all possible conclusions when caring for someone who is mentally ill.

But this, of course, does not always happen. It is possible that your loved one's disturbing behavior will have grown too difficult for you to manage at home, even though you are working with a treatment team. In the face of the mounting challenges, there are other possibilities for you to explore. Hospitalization or skilled nursing facilities may be the only answer for persons who cannot live independently. If they are capable of some level of self-care but cannot live independently, there are halfway houses, residential treatment programs, and board and care facilities. And for those who are able to assume a high level of responsibility and self-care, assisted independent living programs that involve renting cooperatively run apartments or houses may be the answer. In these settings, counselors are available as needed, although they usually are not on the premises twenty-four hours a day. (In the resource section, I list ways to get more information on these options.)

Your caregiving doesn't end here, however. More likely than not, you will visit as much as possible, and though someone else is providing for the physical needs of the one who is ill, you will continue to provide for his or her emotional needs.

According to many who have adult mentally ill family members, there is one other possibility that you have to bear in mind. No matter what you do, or how much you try to provide what is best, the ill one may make decisions that are contrary to your wishes—even leaving home and deciding not to seek treatment, the worst possible scenario. It is important to realize that no matter how hard you try, you cannot always make everything right for a loved one who is suffering from a serious mental illness. You must then come to terms with a difficult situation that has no resolution.

Your caregiving responsibilities may end with death, as they did with Reverend Rex's son Chris. Many individuals express grief at this time, while others experience relief that their loved one's suffering is over—for some it is a guilty relief. Either response (and even both at once) is normal and to be expected.

However you react, you must be aware that you might even experience a sense of loss that the activity of caregiving itself has ended. As burdensome as it can be, caregiving also has the potential to lend meaning and purpose to one's life.

Your Emotional Dilemmas as a Family Caregiver

While you have been spared the physical and mental symptoms of your family member's illness, you may be experiencing many emotions that are difficult to manage.

You may be feeling sadness over the illness of a child, or great personal loss when your spouse, whom you love dearly, can no longer do what he or she was once able to do. The friend, companion, lover, and partner that you once enjoyed may, for all practical purposes, be lost—temporarily or permanently, depending on the severity of the illness.

And you may be frightened. When your family member's symptoms are erratic, you are constantly under the stress of not knowing what to expect. You may find it difficult to plan for the future, or even for daily activities. Your anxiety and helplessness may be painful beyond measure.

Maybe you also feel debilitating guilt about the situation. You worry that you were somehow responsible for the illness, even though you recognize the biological basis of serious mental illness. Or you may worry that you're not doing enough to help the one who is suffering, even though you're already at the end of your rope. Or you feel guilty for the resentment you're experiencing. Or you think that God is punishing you for former transgressions; you might even lose faith in God for having made a good and innocent person suffer so much. Guilt such as this can drain your energy and interfere with your ability to be helpful.

And like some of the respondents in our RCI study, you may feel ambivalent, resentful, angry, trapped, and burdened. Perhaps your family member is ungrateful or physically or emotionally unable to express gratitude or even abusive. How you long to hear those sweet words "Thank you." You are sometimes enraged that recalcitrant family members are unwilling to help. You may wonder when there will be time for your needs.

All of these reactions are normal and to be expected. After all, it's unlikely that having an ill family member would engender happy emotions! Most caregivers experience these feelings every day of their lives. Feelings don't always have to make sense. In order for you to do the best job possible for the one who is ill, it is important for you to acknowledge your emotions, if only to yourself. Feel your pain and grieve for your losses if you must. Whether you like or understand them, these emotions are real and deserve your attention.

To understand your feelings better, ask yourself the following questions:

• Do I feel as if my life is now spinning out of my control?
• Do I feel as if I'm a different person since my family member was diagnosed?
• Do I resent that my previously independent family member has now become dependent on me?
• Am I afraid that others will make derogatory comments about my family member's appearance or condition? Does this keep me from going out more often?
• Do I sometimes wish that I could run away from my situation?
• Do I feel angry:
    —at my family member for constantly needing my attention?
    —at myself for my own limitations?

—at others for their insensitivity or unwillingness to help?

—at the illness itself?

- Have I lost connections with friends and family? Do I feel isolated and alone?
- Do I worry about the impending death of the loved one? Do I sometimes look forward to it with a sense of relief?

If you answered yes to any or all of these questions, do not feel ashamed. This is the normal response for a person in a caregiving role. Now let's see what you can do to ease these troubling feelings.

First you must know that none of these reactions is inappropriate. By acknowledging this, you can avoid the unnecessary pain brought on by guilt for your own anger, frustration, and discouragement.

You may find it useful to list and grieve for the losses you experience. They can be mundane, such as loss of vacation or weekly bridge games; they can be more abstract and all-encompassing, such as lost freedom, privacy, mothering, companionship, or sexuality.

If after noting all that you and the one you care for have lost, you feel like crying, let the tears flow. You're entitled. Crying is a valuable way to release pain, frustration, anger, and grief. Dr. Leonard Felder recommends a weekly cry. "Just like heavy rainfall clears the air and is followed by the sweet sound of birds singing," he writes in his book *When a Loved One Is Ill,* "so does a good cry bathe your insides with a healing release." Dr. Felder encourages caregivers to cry perhaps by watching sad movies, or while taking hot showers, looking at photos of their ill one, or going on long walks near a body of water.[7]

Try to carve some time out of every day that is yours and yours alone. It might make you feel better to weed a small patch in your garden or work a crossword puzzle. Find ways to reduce your stress. An afternoon at the movies with a friend or a walk around the block if you can get away for a while, or even making yourself a simple cup of tea just the way you like it can restore your energy and sense of control, at least for the moment.

In *Helping Yourself Help Others,* I also wrote that you have to be careful how you express your anger. Glowering, stomping around the house, and behaving in a hostile way are rarely effective. And while it's normal to have arguments from time to time, there is little to gain from blasting the ill one or other family members with months of pent-up rage.

More positive ways to vent your rage include exercise, which can help you physically as well as give you a chance to work off the tension and anger you feel; pounding nails into a plank of wood; watching a bruising football game on TV and cheering for your team; or even going out to the car, turning the stereo up high, and screaming as loud as you can!

On the other hand, you might also try meditation and relaxation tapes to help calm your nerves. If you need more help in dealing with your rage, seek out a trusted counselor, perhaps a member of the clergy, or a professional. Don't just let the feelings seethe inside you.

Dealing with Isolation

Sandra Wolfenbarger, a member of our community in southwest Georgia, addressed a conference at the Rosalynn Carter Institute. Sandra's husband had been deeply depressed, and she suffered from isolation. "I had no one I could call and talk to," she told the other family caregivers assembled for the meeting. "I had no one for support. I had no one for advice. We were in a new area. I had no friends. I stood alone.

"We caregivers are going through things," she continued, "and we feel like we're the invisible people. We're the ones who are shouldering the family, we're shouldering the finances, we're responsible for these individuals emotionally, mentally, and physically. Where's our support? We're not professionals. We haven't taken one single course in this field, and yet we're supposed to handle these crises all alone."

Fortunately, Sandra did find help and support for herself. She became the chairperson of the regional affiliate of the National Alliance for the Mentally Ill, and joined the board of directors of the local National Mental Health Association. But her feelings are common among those who care for a family member who has a mental illness.

When you perceive yourself as being alone and in "second place," with no one to talk to or help out, you may feel trapped—literally imprisoned in your own household. These feelings can lead to intense anger and depression, which can further drive away friends and family.

In the RCI survey of family caregivers, we found that respondents rated "linkage with other caregivers" as one of the most pressing, concrete needs. Caregivers need to spend time with other caregivers. They derive much solace from sharing with those in similar situations. It's the best way to fight isolation—to reverse the feeling that "I am the only one" in the world with these problems.[8]

Support groups are the best way to help alleviate the sense of utter aloneness that you may be experiencing. Indeed, they can be crucial for your well-being. They can:

- Help you learn more about your loved one's disorder, including treatment, prognosis, and what the future may hold
- Provide practical suggestions for dealing with hallucinations, delusions, etc., and how to handle crises, such as inappropri-

ate behavior in public, conflicts with law enforcement, and so on

- Provide information about the best community resources and the most responsive professionals
- Create networking connections so that family members who are ill gain access to the best care possible
- Lessen the sense of stigma associated with the illness
- Give you an opportunity to joke and laugh about your circumstances with new friends who really understand and won't judge you
- Give you an opportunity to cry and complain without others urging you to "buck up" or making you feel guilty about your own needs and pain
- Give you a moment to focus on just yourself
- Help you brainstorm solutions to your problems
- Relieve stress and help you feel more in control of your life
- Give you hope as you listen to how others have coped in similar situations

Organizations such as the National Alliance for the Mentally Ill have local support groups. Hospital settings often provide therapeutic groups for patients' family members. Houses of worship may also offer opportunities for sharing. The week before Reverend John Rex delivered the sermon about his son, he showed our video, *Conversations at The Carter Center: Coping with the Stigma of Mental Illness.* In a letter to us, he wrote, "I used that tape last Saturday evening at a potluck dinner/discussion at my fellowship, attended by twenty-two people. The video launched an amazing discussion, during which a number of people shared their own experiences with mental illness, depression, medications, hospitalizations, and so on. . . . It did much good."

If you have access to the Internet, there is a world of information available to you from the various mental health organizations and government agencies. See appendix D for a list of Web sites. You can find the NAMI support group closest to you, and also "chat" via computer with many who find themselves alone in situations similar to yours.

Other community resources can also be helpful. The National Federation of Interfaith Volunteer Caregivers is a not-for-profit organization established in 1984 by the Robert Wood Johnson Foundation, the largest health care foundation in the United States, to promote the ministry of caregiving. Volunteers provide respite for caregivers, transportation to medical appointments, friendly phone calls, home visits, light housekeeping, and other services.

The organization works with coalitions of congregations in all fifty states, the District of Columbia, the Territory of Guam, Puerto Rico, the Virgin Islands, and Canada. Each coalition mobilizes volunteers from diverse congregations within a community. Interfaith Volunteer Caregivers help everyone regardless of age, race, or religion, and they do so without any attempt to proselytize. They see this activity as their ministry.

To illustrate how Interfaith Volunteer Caregivers can help families, executive director Virginia Schiaffino told me about Will, a postman in Washington, D.C. Will's wife, Alicia, had attempted suicide. When she was discharged from the hospital a week before Christmas, Will was told that he could not leave her alone: the holidays are particularly dangerous for people suffering from severe depression.

But Will was unable to take off from work during the busiest mail season of the year. He appealed to his local Interfaith Volunteer Caregivers program for help. The project director responded by organizing teams of trained volunteers to sit with Alicia day and night.

Will could not believe that strangers would give up their Christmas to help him. After all, spending time with someone who is suicidal can be frightening. Moreover, the volunteers were sacrificing hours they would otherwise devote to cooking, shopping, and being with their families. Their acts of kindness strengthened Will, relieved him, and eventually brought him back to the church. They even bolstered Alicia's resolve.

Only you can decide what kind of support suits you best. But please do seek it out. No one should have to go through the experience of caregiving alone. You deserve the comfort of others.

Dealing with Stigma

The powerful stigma of serious mental illness often isolates families from neighbors, relatives, and friends. Families find themselves increasingly alone as others withdraw. They may also hasten their own seclusion by hiding a relative's mental illness from others around them. This self-imposed detachment and secrecy can also contribute to guilt and poor self-esteem. Families may fear being embarrassed by unpredictable behaviors or criticized for their role in caregiving.

The stigma of mental illness often rubs off on caregivers. It seems that no one is interested in their plight. Like Sandra Wolfenbarger, many feel as if no one cares about them. Friends may drop in from time to time, but many feel they are doing so out of a sense of duty—or pity. Or, when others do care, they are sometimes at a loss to know how to behave or respond. Feeling helpless and awkward, they shy away from the situation.

In *Helping Yourself Help Others,* I wrote about a man who complained that friends and relatives had avoided him ever since his son was diagnosed with schizophrenia. "The stigma of a mental disorder causes you to lose many friends," he had said with some bitterness. "Even family back off; they're not around very much. I feel shunned by them. Our friends and family have not been supportive."

And John Rex wrote in his sermon, "There are so many like Chris, so many whose lives are ravaged by mental illness, yet we continue to stigmatize them and their families, to discriminate against them in our health care system, and to abandon them to lives of utter hopelessness. Amazingly, families suffer in silence. People are afraid to speak out, even when speaking out is the only way to gain understanding."

The more stigmatized you feel, the heavier your sense of burden. Allan V. Horwitz and Susan C. Reinhard of Rutgers University studied caregiving burdens among parents and siblings of people with severe mental illness. "It is not just the symptoms and behaviors of mental illnesses that create burden," they wrote. "The burden of caring for a seriously mentally ill child is magnified when caregivers believe their child has a socially stigmatized condition."[9]

You are likely to encounter stigma at almost every turn: with friends, relatives, in outings with your loved one, in looking for housing and employment for him or her, even among mental health professionals. This is a burden that all those who suffer from mental illness and their families experience. I have been told that the best way to handle it is to accept that it will happen . . . and be open about your situation.

That's not to say that it will be easy; it can hurt—but acknowledging it is important. As Rebecca Woolis[10] writes in *When Someone You Love Has a Mental Illness,* because stigma is "based on ignorance and myths, the best antidote is education and first-hand experience. . . . You are in an ideal position to give people some basic information which can lessen fears, dispel misconceptions, and open their hearts to those struggling with mental illness. . . .

"With close friends you might give a more detailed explanation of what has happened and the impact it has had on you and the rest of your family . . . with people you don't know very well, or with neighbors, you may want to give a very abridged version. You can assure them that [your ill family member] is not dangerous and tell them that they ought to just say hello if they see him outside, even if he appears to be talking to himself. . . .

"You may want to tell [people] that, in many ways, a mental illness is like dealing with diabetes or cancer. . . . Thus by comparing mental illness with cancer or diabetes, you may give people a better idea of what you are going through and how they can be supportive of you."

She goes on to say that educating your friends, colleagues, and relatives puts another burden on you, "but this is one I strongly encourage you to embrace, at least for a few important people in your life. Otherwise you will find yourself in the all-too-common position of feeling further isolated and resentful of friends and relatives. Deciding you cannot talk to anyone about one of the most significant parts of your life is bound to take its toll."

I want to add that by educating others you will not only be helping yourself, but you will be helping countless individuals; you will be contributing to overcoming the stigma that causes untold suffering.

Dealing with Burnout

Burnout is the feeling of having reached the limits of one's endurance and ability to cope. It results from the combination of emotional dilemmas including feelings of helplessness, guilt, lack of appreciation for one's efforts, family discord, and isolation. Add to that the urgency and tension caused by too many demands on one's strength, resources, time, and energy and it becomes clear why many caregivers experience this sense of utter depletion.

A woman wrote to me about friends—a husband and wife—who were struggling with the husband's depression:

> His wife is exhausted and nearly at her wits' end. They are in terrible debt due to medical bills, and she is isolated and completely demoralized. She feels so helpless and overwhelmed that she has thought of divorcing him to save herself, but she fears that this would surely cause him to kill himself.

The wife is obviously suffering from burnout. Unfortunately, this is a common occurrence among caregivers, whether the one they are caring for is suffering from a physical or mental illness. In our study at the Rosalynn Carter Institute, we found that about half of those surveyed believed they were probably suffering from burnout, and 85 percent complained of feeling "just plain exhausted" at the end of the day.

According to clinical psychologist and burnout expert Dr. Herbert J. Freudenberger, physical symptoms of burnout can include headaches, insomnia, backaches, lethargy, lingering colds, gastrointestinal upsets, and cardiovascular problems. Burnout also has emotional components. Caregivers may find themselves feeling frustrated and angry, empty or sad, pessimistic, resentful, insecure, or depressed. These are all expected reactions to feeling stressed beyond one's ability to cope.

Burnout can also be dangerous. Many caregivers who receive inadequate assistance or who cannot locate others with similar problems may become the casualties of the future. Some become so overwhelmed by the burdens of caring for one who is mentally ill that they seek to escape into work or hobbies, leaving the sick one all the more alone. Others may turn to alcohol or drugs to assuage their pain, thus becoming even more incapacitated.

As mentioned earlier, peer support groups are an excellent way for you to revitalize your energy and avoid these kind of situations. There are also other strategies for avoiding burnout:

1. *Listen to friends.* The first step in resolving burnout is recognizing that you are suffering from it. Caregivers should be open to others' observations. If friends have noticed a change in your behavior or demeanor, don't contradict them without first taking a minute to evaluate whether what they are saying is true.

2. *Educate yourself.* "Somebody needs to give caregivers a road map," said one participant in our RCI study. It's natural to feel bewildered by it all. But understanding the course of the disorder, the possibility of relapse, the recommended treatments, the side effects of medications, and all the other complexities of your family member's illness can help you anticipate and plan for the future. It can also reduce your feelings of helplessness and prepare you in advance for dealing with crises. You might seek out additional, specific information from professionals as well as from books and organizations and from the Internet.

3. *Keep a journal.* Dr. Freudenberger suggests that caregivers keep a "Burnout Log" to document daily events that create stress in their lives. After several weeks, you will be able to identify and then draw some conclusions about what aspects of your role you find the most difficult. You may then be able to devise some solutions. For example, in keeping the journal, you may realize how long it has been since you allowed yourself time for a walk . . . or for reading an exciting novel when you are feeling oppressed by the ill one's persistently pessimistic mood.

4. *Maintain friendships.* Even though you may be feeling miserable, it's important that you not isolate yourself from those who can provide support or just a distraction. Studies have shown that people who have friends have a stronger immune system and live longer than those who don't!

5. *Preserve routines.* So often, when mental illness strikes, family members feel out of control. The unpredictability of the illness can wreak havoc on one's sense of stability. Although none of us is in control of everything, it can be comforting and reassuring to retain and maintain as much routine as is reasonable.

Having dinner at 6:00 P.M. each evening, going to church every Sunday, or watching a favorite TV show every day are all simple ways of maintaining a sense of control. Routines can create structure and a feeling of safety.

By the same token, try not to abandon hobbies and other activities that have always given you pleasure. You may need to feed your soul in order to be available to the ill one. By continuing to participate in activities you enjoy, you will have more energy to bring to the caregiving relationship.

6. *Maintain a life outside the caregiving role.* Even though a loved one may be suffering, it's wise for you to remember that you and other well family members are separate people who are entitled to enjoy your own lives. In addition to continuing with your hobbies, you might consider developing new skills. Attend seminars or classes that promote personal and professional growth to prevent the caregiving role from enveloping you. Some caregivers find regular swimming useful since it provides exercise and solitude. Others find photography a good hobby. You can record happy times with your mentally ill family member, and also add beauty to your days by photographing flowers or budding trees or animals in the yard.

7. *Learn relaxation techniques.* Some people find meditation and yoga helpful. Others use biofeedback to relieve stress. It is important to enjoy a relaxing outlet: exercising, listening to music, gardening, reading a good book, sewing, taking a walk, or just napping. Some individuals need to vent their frustrations. Exercise and journal writing can release excess anger and tension before they reach the breaking point.

8. *Let go.* No one person can do it all. Acknowledge that as a human being you have limitations just like everyone else. Allow others to help you and delegate responsibilities. Practice asking for help and saying no once in a while. Lower your expectations and tolerate things that might not get done perfectly—the dishes need not be washed after every meal. Prioritize tasks and learn to manage your time.

Sometimes it's helpful to be passive. Allow yourself to feel replenished from others' gestures—a card, a kind word left on the answering machine, a pat on the arm. Listening to music, attending religious services, or watching a favorite video can also help.

9. *Take care of your own health.* Recent research has shown that stressful situations can encourage smoking, drinking, overeating, or other unhealthy practices. If you ignore your own health, and become depleted and exhausted, you won't be of much help to the one you are caring for. So be sure to eat well and get enough exercise and sleep. Exercise is an excellent way to maintain health and reduce stress. Even if you can't get to the gym regularly, an aerobics video, a brisk walk, or a stint pulling weeds can do wonders in restoring energy. And always seek medical care for any physical problems you may have.

10. *Rely on a sense of humor.* What better time to laugh than when the situation looks bleak? A good chuckle can get most of us through the worst of times. Peer support groups can be quite

useful in this regard. You will probably have to look for the humor in daily activities, but try to make light of difficult situations and laugh about them—if you can! Your tasks will be easier.

11. *Seek professional help.* You may benefit from seeing a counselor who specializes in stress reduction or who works with families dealing with mental illnesses. It may help to discuss negative feelings about the ill loved one and the caregiving experience in a safe environment. A counselor can help you let go of unrealistic expectations and can teach you new coping strategies.

12. *Seek spiritual renewal.* The participants in our caregiving study at the RCI found solace in their faith, so a faith congregation may be your primary source of help. Religious services, conversations with clergy, or individual worship can help to alleviate your stress and give you strength and inspiration.

Another Story of Hope

In his memoir *Darkness Visible,* William Styron applauds the all-important role of the family caregiver, especially in the case of depression. "A tough job, this" he writes. "Calling 'Chin up!' from the safety of the shore to a drowning person is tantamount to insult, but it has been shown over and over again that if the encouragement is dogged enough—and the support equally committed and passionate—the endangered one can nearly always be saved. . . . It may require on the part of friends, lovers, family, and admirers an almost religious devotion to persuade the sufferers of life's worth, which is so often in conflict with a sense of their own worthlessness, but such devotion has prevented countless suicides."[11]

Stuart Perry,[12] an employee at an auto parts store and a survivor of depression, is the recipient of just such dogged devotion, and he talked about it at one of our RCI conferences.

Pointing to photographs of his wife, daughter, and in-laws, Stuart said, "That's my backbone. Because of them, I'm able to stand before you today." Characterizing himself as "a man who didn't even know who he was" when in the grips of his illness, he described the love and support he received from his family. "My family has been behind me one hundred percent, and I'm really thankful to them."

Then he went on to explain. "I lost my father to depression in 1981. He committed suicide, and I saw it right before my eyes. Eight years later, I woke up one morning in a depression—I had hallucinations, the whole nine yards. . . ." He passed around photographs of himself while he was deeply depressed—unkempt, bushy hair and beard—so that we could appreciate how far he had come.

"I'm trying to go out to the community now to educate folks so what happened to my father won't happen to anyone else. I'm very fortunate that the same thing didn't happen to me. One of the main reasons is because of my family. They picked up on all of the signs of depression that I had no idea about and helped save my life."

Stuart spoke with a great deal of humor and affection about his family and the encouragement he had received from them. He said that he and his wife, Pam, had been up since 4:00 A.M. because he was so nervous about addressing our group. She had reassured him by saying, "Even if you bomb there today, we'll still be waiting for you here at home."

Then he regaled us with stories about his father-in-law. "When I was so sick, my father-in-law put his arm around me and said, 'Son, it doesn't matter to me what you do in life. I don't care if you're rich. I don't care if you're poor. But you try. That's all I want you to do. You just try.'

"We talked for a long time that day," Stuart continued. "My father-in-law said, 'Tell you what I'm gonna do. You keep on going to those meetings with your counselor and you keep taking that medicine. Me and your mother-in-law are going to get your family a new place to live.' So they went out and bought us a real nice place. I'm very proud of it. It has a pretty yard. Then he said, 'Tell you what I'm gonna do. I'm gonna buy you a lawn mower.' He didn't buy me one of those riding lawn mowers but one you have to push. He said, 'I got you two acres of land out there. I want you to push that thing.' "

This brought laughter from the audience. Stuart went on. "They got me two acres of Bahia grass. You cut it today, and you cut it tomorrow.

"Then my uncle came out and he said, 'Do you know what you've got to do? You've got to put some nitrogen on that grass.' So I went to the store and got me some nitrogen. I put it on the grass, and you know what? I thought I was hallucinating again. Before I got to the top of the hill, the Bahia grass was two feet tall behind me!"

Then, bringing out an enormous trophy, he said, "One thing that came out of this is now I walk a lot of marathons. I came in third place in the Americus Walk-America race!" He brandished the award overhead to loud applause.

"I'm a lucky person," he continued. "I see people every day who are afraid to ask for help but want to ask for help. There's that stigma. 'I'm crazy. How do I ask for help?' " Clearly, Stuart was able to overcome the stigma. He not only received help from his family but now gives it to others who are struggling to understand their loved one's illness.

He closed his remarks by reciting the lyrics to a song sung by Celine Dion, "Because You Loved Me,"[13] changing a single word to dedicate it to all those who had helped him overcome depression—especially his family:

> For all the times you stood by me,
> For all the truth that you made me see,
> For all the joy that you brought to my life,
> For all the wrongs that you made right,
> For every dream that you made come true
> For all the love I found in you,
> I'll be forever thankful, caregivers.
> You're the ones who helped me up and never let me fall;
> You're the ones who saw me through it all.

When he was finished, there were tears and a standing ovation.

❧

I hope the information in this chapter has given you some ideas, information, and concrete advice that will assist you in carrying out your role as a caregiver and help you feel not quite so alone. You are essential to your loved one's good mental and physical health. You belong to a special category of unsung heroes and heroines who deserve support, services, and praise for your extraordinary personal sacrifices and the contributions you make not only to your loved one, but also to our society.

Chapter 12

Advocating for the Mentally Ill

During our April 1996 Conversations at The Carter Center, the subject of stigma surfaced once more during the question and answer period. And, in his inimitable way, actor Rod Steiger sought to define it simply and succinctly. "Stigma is a prejudice," he bellowed from his seat in response to a query. "A prejudice. Like a racial prejudice or a religious prejudice. That's what you're dealing with—a prejudice—and it's based on instincts."

Then he went on to explain. "Look," he said, "you have a purple man and a yellow man going through the woods. They each think that they are the only man on earth. They *are* the only two, but they don't know it; they haven't seen each other. The yellow one goes hunting, he turns the corner, and Jesus, there's a purple man! His instincts—not his mind—will put him on the defensive. . . . [The purple man] is something unknown. That's what makes stigma tough to fight, because part of it is instinctive. . . . And that's why knowledge takes that fear away."

In the introduction to *Stigma and Mental Illness,* my friend Paul Jay Fink,[1] chairman of the Department of Psychiatry at Albert Einstein Medical Center in Philadelphia, defines stigma associated with mental illnesses as the marginalization and ostracism of individuals because they are mentally ill. And stigma is characterized by Erving Goffman, eminent social psychologist,[2] as a state of being disqualified from social acceptance—being "deeply discredited."

Why have those with mental illnesses been stigmatized—ostracized by society, discredited, and disgraced? Perhaps Rod is right. Their behavior or appearance seems different to those of us who are not ill, and therefore is threatening. Mental illnesses can be complex, and individuals suffering from them can present us with bizarre symptoms that frighten and distress us. We instinctively fear what we do not know.

During my childhood, the word "cancer" was never spoken out loud. It was a deadly and mysterious disease that was feared, and people suffering from it were shunned. I remember when Jimmy's father was diagnosed in the early 1950s. He had been ill for some time, and after an exploratory operation, when it was discovered that he had cancer, he somehow knew. He never asked what the doctors found, and until his death, the word *cancer* was never uttered in his presence.

Today, after years of research and public education, we recognize cancer as an illness that is challenging to patients and their physicians, but is no longer a cause for shame or discrimination.

Just as with this and other illnesses that have been feared—leprosy, tuberculosis, epilepsy—I look forward to the day when mental illness is understood and accepted as a challenging illness, but without the negative perceptions.

A Short History of Stigma

Stigma toward those suffering from mental disorders dates back through recorded history. The word *stigma* itself comes from ancient Greek, meaning to mark someone, in those days most likely with a tattoo or other brand. Even then, "madness," although viewed as caused by capricious gods, was a source of shame. According to Bennett Simon,[3] professor of psychiatry at Cambridge Hospital in Cambridge, Massachusetts, in ancient Greek society "mental illness, especially if chronic, was regarded at best as undesirable and at worst as requiring that afflicted persons be shunned, locked up, or probably on rare occasions, put to death."

Even in more modern times, mental illnesses were thought to be caused by possession by the devil. According to Norman Dain, professor of history at Rutgers University, "The traditional belief among Christians that madness is often a punishment visited by God on the sinner predominated in American society during the 17th century and remained quite influential thereafter."[4] No wonder mentally ill individuals were confined—chained, humiliated, and abused—in squalid institutions (often jails) for their entire lives. They were seen as deserving punishment.

Pennsylvania Hospital was one of the first general hospitals in colonial America to admit "lunatics," but the abuse continued. Among other ignoble acts there, the public was allowed to come on weekends and view the "lunatics"—for a small fee! In response, Friends Hospital in Philadelphia, which I visited several years ago on its 175th anniversary, was established by the Quakers to provide "moral treatment to mentally ill patients"—which it still does today.

With this kind of past, we can easily understand why there is stigma associated with mental illness.

Stigma and the Media

Kathy Cronkite opened her remarks during our Conversations at The Carter Center program with a challenge for the media.

"It turns out," she said, "that the Unabomber and I take the same medication. I don't know what it means that he takes it, but I know it must be important because the news media reported it. The news media chose to report that fact, along with a handful of items such as bomb parts and hit lists from over three hundred articles that were found in his cabin. Unfortunately, all too often we see these sorts of reports that may serve to further stigmatize the ill and to further frighten people away from what may be lifesaving medication.

"I remember I was in New York when a bomb exploded in a subway there, and a tabloid headline read shortly thereafter 'Mad Bomber! Was Prozac to Blame?' The man had, in fact, been taking an antidepressant. Here's a headline I'd like to see: 'CEO of Major Corporation Announces New Factory, Hires Thousands! Is Prozac to Blame?' " (And I've always wanted to see a sitcom on TV starring a CEO who has overcome a mental illness and is heading a highly successful business!)

Kathy is right, of course. The news and entertainment media have enormous influence on how we perceive those who are mentally ill. One study found that almost all Americans learn what they know about psychiatric illnesses from television,[5] and those portrayals are hardly ever positive or accurate. While less than 3 percent of mentally ill patients have the potential for violence, 77 percent of those depicted on prime-time television are presented as dangerous.[6]

Other media can be just as demeaning. A few years ago I visited Rome, Georgia, a city that has a rather large psychiatric hospital. I was dismayed to learn of the crude jokes on the radio about patients in the hospital. Even ads can be hurtful. In the fall of 1997, there were several promotional spots for the television program *Frasier* that were offensive. One, for example, showed a man repeatedly washing his hands as the bar of soap grew smaller while the voice-over announced, "Get a new obsession . . . watch *Frasier.*" After this advertisement appeared on TV, I received numerous letters from mentally ill people saying "We've been hurt and offended."

Even psychiatrists are not immune from prejudicial portrayals in the media. Steven Sharfstein,[7] a psychiatrist with whom I have worked closely during and since the White House years, has said, "The psychiatrist is often seen, because we have the responsibility of treating people who are mentally ill, as somehow not being quite right ourselves. . . . It's always very refreshing for me to see a film where a psychiatrist is portrayed as a humane and competent person, such as in *Ordinary People,* compared to the way the psychiatrist was portrayed in *Dressed to Kill,* where he was a homicidal maniac."

But *Ordinary People* is the exception. Of the hundreds of movies in which psychiatrists or psychiatric hospitals have been depicted, we need only think of *One Flew over the Cuckoo's Nest* to understand how negatively they can be characterized. And psychiatrists have been variously stereotyped as "the libidinous lecher," "the eccentric buffoon," "the evil-minded doctor," "the unempathic cold fish."[8] Who would want to see such a doctor?

With these images in mind I have been to Hollywood twice, once when Jimmy was president and again since we have been home, to meet with screenwriters, producers, and directors of movies and television programs to impress upon them the need for sensitivity—and accuracy—in their portrayals of mentally ill people.

Stereotyping and sensationalism in the media reinforce the myth that those who have mental illnesses are dangerous. And as Dr. William Dubin of the Philadelphia Psychiatric Center and Paul Fink point out in *Stigma and Mental Illness,* "On the rare occasion when a former mental patient does commit a violent crime, no reporter is interested in the failures of the mental health treatment system that has often allowed these patients to go for long periods of time untreated and, in many instances, to be forced out of hospital settings into the community against the recommendations of psychiatrists."[9]

Fortunately, this is beginning to change, to a great extent as a result of the family-consumer movement, national organizations, and other advocates who are making the elimination of stigma their top priority.

The Consequences of Stigma

In 1972, Senator George McGovern, the Democratic candidate for president, selected Senator Thomas Eagleton of Missouri as his vice presidential running mate.

Soon after, however, word was leaked to the McGovern campaign and eventually to the press that Senator Eagleton had had a mental illness. Eagleton held a press conference during which he admitted to having been "voluntarily" hospitalized three times in the previous twelve years for "nervous exhaustion."

Although Senator McGovern initially expressed confidence in his running mate, and Eagleton's colleagues in Congress applauded his abilities despite his earlier bouts with depression, donations to the Democratic party dropped sharply after the news conference. And a scant two weeks after he was chosen, Senator Eagleton became the first U.S. vice presidential nominee to withdraw from candidacy, a victim of the stigma associated with mental illness.

What are the consequences of stigma? They can be many and far-reaching. As in the case of Tom Eagleton, it can ruin careers and aspirations. And after Kathy Cronkite and Rod Steiger made their presentations at The Carter Center, person after person rose to tell how their lives had been affected.

"I almost didn't come tonight," said one young woman, "because I thought I'd cry through the whole thing. But the compulsion to be with and look at somebody who really understood where I came from was really overwhelming.

"My family disappeared." She turned to Kathy. "I remember reading that your husband supported you, and I prayed that that miracle would somehow come to me too, but it didn't. I asked my husband if he would come with me tonight and he said, 'I've had enough education for a while, thank you very much.' "

Then a mother took the microphone to tell of her experience. "When my son was eighteen, he was a student at one of the best universities in the country. He went in and three weeks after he was in that university, he was psychotic, in the psychiatric unit of the local community hospital. And during the three weeks he was in that hospital, he got not one phone call, not one card, not one flower, not one visit from anyone in that university. His only visitors were his family.

"At the same time there were students there who had been in an automobile accident. Their rooms were full of flowers, the students were in and out, the faculty was there. My son was abandoned . . . now thirteen or fourteen years later he has recovered, he's paying his taxes, he's working. But as a mother, I will never forget the difference between how the boys and girls with the physical illnesses on that campus were treated and how my son was treated."

And another. "I'm back at work; I've been at work since January. I had to lie to get my job because I didn't dare tell them what I had been through. I had to create a story about my daughter having ADD (attention deficit disorder). I've been a successful professional for eleven years, but that would not have mattered."

These stories illustrate the effect of stigma on family relationships, social networks, and employment. Yet one of the saddest consequences of stigma to me is that so many people suffer needlessly. Fear of being labeled mentally ill keeps them from seeking diagnosis and effective treatment.

Take the case of obsessive-compulsive disorder (OCD), which for years was thought to be an extremely rare condition, affecting one in every two thousand people. This statistic was derived from the number of people who visited psychiatric clinics. But when the National Institute of Mental Health began contacting a random sample of U.S. households and institutions, they discovered that one in forty Americans suffers from the disorder, not one in two thousand.

"At first we thought this was a false finding," says Jeffrey M. Schwartz of the UCLA Neuropsychiatric Institute, "but it's not. Insight is preserved in people with OCD. They know the condition is embarrassing, so they hide it . . . [and when they do] and don't seek treatment, their symptoms will only get worse. There is no disease in psychiatry where it's more evident that stigma has prevented people from getting treatment than OCD."

Those who suffer cannot escape the consequences of stigma. They are reflected in our laws—zoning laws, insurance laws, discriminatory Medicare and Medicaid rules and housing regulations—and in funding for research and treatment for mental illnesses.

I feel the same as one mother who wrote to me when she was trying to locate her homeless son who suffers from schizophrenia: "I cannot grasp the *whys* of the laws that apply to mentally ill people who have never asked to be that way."

The net effect of the consequences of stigma is untold suffering and a great loss of human potential.

Stigma and the Insurance Industry

One area in which the consequences of stigma take a particularly high toll on families is that of insurance coverage. Over 95 percent of all health insurance plans discriminate against people with mental illness through higher copayments, arbitrary treatment limits, or outright exclusions.[10]

For years, I and many others have been lobbying for what is called "parity." Parity simply means that mental illnesses should receive the same health insurance benefits as physical illnesses—in other words, there should be fairness in mental health coverage. Mental illnesses should have the same deductibles, the same copayments, the same annual and lifetime limits, and arbitrary treatment limits should be outlawed.

Lower benefits for these illnesses result in inadequate care or financial disaster for those afflicted and their families. Sherry, a young woman with mental illness, points up the trauma of the lack of parity. Her situation was a typical one. While her insurance company covered 80 to 100 percent of her regular medical bills, it covered only 50 percent of her mental health bills, with a very low lifetime cap and restrictions on the number of days she could be hospitalized for reasons pertaining to mental illness. In a letter to me, Sherry wrote,

> My doctor has had to release me from the hospital before I was ready on one occasion because my days were up. . . . Another time, because I could not afford the 50% co-payment, I put off seeking help until the last moment. I was told that if I had waited another 24 hours, my doctor would have had no choice but to commit me.

Why should Sherry have to suffer so, for lack of adequate insurance coverage?

The main objection to parity is the belief that insurance costs will escalate dramatically. The fact is that it is much more cost-effective to diagnose and treat mental illnesses in the early stages than to allow them to develop into serious problems that can require long-term hospitalization. In addition, as I mentioned in chapter 5, evidence is now accumulating to show that comprehensive mental health coverage actually reduces the total cost of health care over a period of time.

In 1994, Betty Ford and I met with key congressional leaders to advocate that mental illness and addiction be included on a par with physical illness in the proposed national health care reform initiative. Despite the fact that reform has not gone forward, the collective efforts of the mental health community were instrumental in the passage of a new law, the Health Insurance Portability and Accountability Act of 1996, which abolished the unfair lifetime caps—such as the one that plagued my correspondent, Sherry. Many changes are occurring at state levels. Nondiscrimination legislation is being introduced in state legislatures, and mental health advocates are organizing, as someone has said, from "Vermont to Hawaii." And we will continue our efforts at the state level and with Congress until these illnesses are adequately covered in all health insurance plans.

I have always believed that if insurance coverage made no distinction among illnesses, a lot of the stigma of the mental illnesses would fade away. The fact that they were covered would make them acceptable. Creating a health care system that reflects parity acknowledges the need to see people as whole human beings, and it recognizes the worth of every person, regardless of his or her disability.

Changing Public Attitudes

The fear and misunderstanding of mental illnesses and emotional problems are deeply ingrained in our society, and changing attitudes takes time. I know this well, after having worked on this issue for more than twenty-five years. Yet, though negative perceptions still persist, some progress is being made as a result of a number of developments.

Because the media is so powerful in influencing attitudes, there has been a recognition of the need for cooperation between mental health advocates and the people who work for the media. At the same time we have seen the rise of new organizations made up of consumers and their families—not only because of the need to change attitudes and educate people, but also because of *hope,* brought about by new knowledge and the discovery of new treatments.

When Jimmy and I left the White House in 1981, the National Alliance for the Mentally Ill was little more than an idea. It has since become one of the most influential and effective movements in mental health history—a movement made up of many thousands of parents, siblings, spouses, and other relatives or friends who have come together to work for better care for their loved ones. This was the beginning of families and consumers "coming out of the closet"—and once begun, it exploded. Indeed, many organizations consisting solely of consumers have also grown to be a powerful advocacy voice at national, state, and local levels.

I remember going to NAMI's annual meeting in 1987. I was to speak after dinner, and wanting to be accurate I asked my dinner partner if the figure I had for the number of chapters over the country was correct. When he looked at my speech notes, he said, "Mrs. Carter, these are last week's figures, and they're old!" At that time, he told me they were adding one new chapter every thirty-six hours, one person every six minutes!

From my earliest attempts to help, I have thought that the best thing I could do was focus attention on the issue of mental illness, in an effort to decrease stigma. In the early 1970s, when any progress was so difficult, just talking about it was important—bringing the subject out in the open, trying to make it an acceptable topic of conversation. I thought that if I and other public figures talked about it, we could demonstrate it was not a taboo subject, and this might encourage those who suffer to be more willing to seek help.

Our first symposium at The Carter Center in 1985 was organized around stigma, because I feel so strongly about it. Again in 1988 we focused on mental illness and the media, bringing together representatives from the media and entertainment communities with the mental health community. As a follow-up to this symposium, we developed and distributed a list of suggestions that could be used when portraying mentally ill people and their families, facilities and services, and mental health professionals (see pages 245–47).

As the advocacy movement has grown, there has been a great increase in anti-stigma activities. Many national organizations run education campaigns that include public service announcements, advertisements, 800 numbers, and pamphlets and awareness guides.

Many have also developed "media watch" programs, in which members of organizations take turns monitoring news broadcasts, TV and radio programs, and advertisements. When they see insensitive depictions and hear language that hurts mentally ill people, they notify other members and mount a letter-writing campaign. I received a "Stigma Alert," for example, from the national Stigma Clearinghouse in New York and one from the Anxiety Disorders Association of America when the *Frasier* television program promotional spot was shown. Each asked that I contact my local broadcaster if the ad ran in my area. I have joined in many of these efforts—once writing a letter to Dan Rather about a story on the evening news that horribly misrepresented mentally ill people.

The month of May has become National Mental Health Month sponsored by the National Mental Health Association, one of the oldest and most effective advocacy organizations. This special month is observed by almost all organizations, providers, and advocacy groups nationwide. State governors proclaim the month, and community clubs and organizations conduct educational programs and sponsor events to increase public awareness about mental illnesses and about the progress being made in treatment and research. And in the early 1980s, Congress declared the first full week of every October Mental Illness Awareness Week. One of the many activities that take place during this week is National Depression Screening Day, with hundreds of thousands of people visiting their local hospitals, shopping malls, schools, and libraries to participate in medical screenings for depression. There is also a National Anxiety Disorders Screening Day in early May, which has been very successful.

Another important trend of the last decade is that we, the American public, have become very conscious of health issues in general. Now there are regular segments on health-related subjects in many different types of media. As I was writing this book, for example, one night I saw a health segment on ABC News that focused on phobia. It was well done and examined the problem in depth. A man was interviewed about his experiences with the illness, then the symptoms were listed on the screen, and a doctor explained how someone could be treated. This kind of program offers invaluable help in educating people and helping them recognize symptoms that they or loved ones may be experiencing—and it helps in overcoming stigma. The subject of mental illness is coming up more and more on talk shows, radio programs, and in news stories and magazine articles.

I believe this reflects the great interest of people in learning more about the illnesses and the growing willingness to discuss and be identified with the issue—I hope! It also shows the impact of mental health advocates and organizations.

Historically, advocacy for mentally ill citizens has grown out of the experiences of someone—or a few people—who have been affected by the illness. The National Mental Health Association had its beginning when a man named Clifford Beers experienced a mental breakdown. After his recovery in the early 1900s, he devoted himself to the study and advancement of mental health. And NAMI grew out of the experiences of families who had loved ones stricken with mental illness: When Carol and Jim Howe, who had two mentally ill sons, met Dr. Agnes Hatfield, a scholar with a mentally ill family member, she had already begun gathering together others with the same problem. They joined in forming a group and soon learned that other such groups were spontaneously forming across the land.

Terrence Caster, a prominent San Diego, California, real estate developer, shares the feeling and ambition of these individuals. He has developed a project called Erasing the Stigma of Mental Illness (ETS) that he hopes will become a nationwide organization. His actions have grown out of experiences with a family member who was incarcerated after an acute episode of illness led to a violent incident. "My family member had been having problems for a number of years with alcohol and drugs," Terrence told me, "but we skirted the thing and we didn't know what to do about it."

The "thing" the Casters had skirted was schizophrenia. But they were forced to confront it. "We saw up close how terribly painful mental illness is," he said. "The pain and suffering is unimaginable . . . and extremely costly. We had to go through a long court trial. And seeing our family member's hands in handcuffs behind his back, and in the small cages. . . . It was a terrible, terrible thing.

"Once we had seen how much pain there was in this illness, my wife and I said, 'My God, we should do something about it. There must be millions of other people out there who are experiencing this terrible thing.' "

Terrence wanted to create an entity that would help others so that they wouldn't have to hit bottom, as his family member did. Thus was born ETS, an educational program designed to increase the understanding of mental illness and encourage its early treatment. The program, endorsed by the American Psychiatric Association, provides tapes, videos, and speakers to civic clubs and other organizations. And they are having an impact. Terrence reported, "For the last five years, I don't think there has ever been a speaking engagement where the speaker hasn't reported back to us that at the conclusion of the talk people come up and say, 'You know, that really hit home. I have a sister, brother, mother, daughter . . .' All of them say, 'This is good news; I feel better about it; there is hope.' "

And what of Terrence's family member? He was properly diagnosed while incarcerated and begun on a low dose of medication that has made a world of difference. Terrence told me, "He has been five years clean and sober, working every day."

All of these efforts, together, are making a difference. Coalitions have developed that are having a political impact, as was seen in the public debates during health care reform, and in the enactment of legislation improving insurance coverage for mental illnesses.

Recent polls have shown that people's opinions about mental illness are also being positively influenced. For example, in September 1996 our mental health program at The Carter Center helped draft questions for a statewide poll in Georgia. We were all excited—and gratified—by the results:

- 94.8 percent of those polled believed that people with mental illness can be helped with proper treatment
- 90.8 percent believed that health insurance policies should provide the same coverage for mental illnesses as they do for physical ones
- 82.4 percent would support a candidate for elected office who had been treated for mental illness if they believed that person was the best for the position

But, in answer to another question, 48.9 percent would not want their employer to know that they were seeking treatment for a mental illness. Stigma!

What You Can Do About Stigma

There is reason for cautious optimism, both because of the actions that many are taking to reverse the injustices that those with mental illnesses have long endured, and because of the polls that are beginning to show some signs of understanding and acceptance by the public. Yet we still have a long way to go in overcoming the stigma. It will take all of us working together to make significant progress.

What can *you* do to fight stigma? There are many actions you can take—at home, in your schools and community, and on a national level.

Personal/Family

• Talk to your children about mental illness. Explain that mental health is as vital a part of total health as physical health.

• When you see a depiction of a mentally ill person on television or in the movies, make it a topic of family discussion. Is that depiction accurate? Why or why not?

• Talk about stigma with your children. Explain how it is a form of prejudice. Discuss the incorrect stereotypes of mentally ill people as violent or dangerous.

• Consider taking your children to visit a community center or group home for people who are mentally ill (assuming you have the approval of people living there); what we don't know, we often misjudge. However, be sure to prepare them well before the trip. A friend of mine recalled how she was frightened when her school choir performed a Christmas concert at a nearby mental health facility. "No one told us that many of the patients would be catatonic or behave oddly, but that they were non-violent and appreciative of our efforts, even if they couldn't show it. As a result, we were all terrified and confused," she said.

• Use "people first" language, such as referring to "a person with schizophrenia," *not* "a schizophrenic."

• Never use discriminatory slang such as "crazy" to describe people or situations, and correct your children when they use such derogatory language.

In Schools

• If mental health—including warning signs of depression and other mental illness—is not part of the school health curriculum, write to the principal, school board, or superintendent to get it included. In my conversations with early childhood educators, I have been told that this discussion should probably start at about the fifth grade, when children are developmentally able to deal with abstract thinking.

• Advocate that students learn about the disability rights movement and the Americans with Disabilities Act (ADA)—including the rights of mentally disabled people—just as they learn about civil rights and women's rights.

• If you hear of a mentally disabled student who is being stigmatized, discuss with teachers and the principal what actions can be taken to stop the situation and educate the student body.

• Ask the teacher to correct the use of "crazy" and other derogatory slang.

In the Community

• Join your local branch of the NMHA or NAMI, Anxiety Disorders Association of America, or other advocacy organization. There is power in numbers.

• Write to editors of local newspapers and television and radio stations that publish or broadcast expressions or descriptions that may demean someone suffering from a mental illness, or if they have demeaning and unbalanced coverage of mental health issues.

• Also, write to them encouraging programs that educate the public about these illnesses and encourage them to include stories about mentally ill people who have been successfully treated and are now active, productive citizens in the community.

• Contact the Media Watch programs of your local advocacy organizations.

• Point out to store managers displays that use discriminatory advertising.

• Learn more about community centers and group homes for mentally ill people. Educate your neighbors and friends about them; support them by volunteering, by contributions, or by lobbying for laws that help them; vote for candidates who support them; speak up at town meetings; and do what you can to eliminate prejudice against them.

Nationally

• Contact radio and TV stations not only to report inappropriate references to mental illness, but to advocate for more—and more balanced—coverage of mental illness.

• Write to publishers of books, newspapers, and magazines, pointing out inappropriate references to or demeaning descriptions of people afflicted with mental illness.

• Vote for candidates with strong mental health platforms.

• Urge politicians with personal histories of mental illness or others with mental illness to step forward with their stories to help destigmatize the issues. Write letters to the editors of national magazines and major newspapers to voice your support of those who do.

• Join and support national lobbying organizations such as NMHA and NAMI.

• Write to your senators and members of Congress, advocating for parity in the coverage of mental illness.

What We're Doing About Stigma at The Carter Center

In our mental health program at The Carter Center, we have several anti-stigma initiatives currently under way. The Conversation at The Carter Center program with Kathy Cronkite and Rod Steiger, which we have developed into an excellent videotape, is part of that effort. The video has been shown on PBS and is available to the public through The Carter Center. It is also available for viewing as a public service video in Blockbuster Video stores across the country.

Our latest initiative is a fellowship program for journalists. Each year, for a period of five years, we are supporting five journalists to study selected topics regarding mental health issues. We want to add to the number of journalists who are interested in these issues and who can report and promote accurate information about mental health and mental illness in the media.

In the planning stage is an Anti–Stigma Task Force made up of people representing business, education, health care, the media, and the religious community. We want to see how each sector can help those it reaches. How can businesses, for instance, profit by providing mental health coverage for their employees? How can clergy help their congregations overcome stigma? What will it take for health educators to teach that mental illnesses are diseases just like any other? Each sector can make a difference, and we want to explore the ways they can help.

We also continue to distribute the list of suggestions that can be used by media for accurately portraying families, facilities, services, and professionals who care for mentally ill people. The list is available from The Carter Center for media or for advocates who would like to distribute it to their local media.

The Carter Center Mental Illnesses and Entertainment Media Depiction Suggestions

Depicting Families of People with Mental Illnesses

- Emphasize that blaming family members for a child's mental illness is incorrect.

- Include in stories the painful, often devastating impact of mental illness on family members.
- Have characters mention community and self-help services that are available to help them cope with the impact of mental illness.
- Show positive living relationships between family members and people with mental illnesses as part of some stories and show that there is really hope for healing and recovery.

Depicting Professionals Who Work with People with Mental Illnesses

- Show therapists as human beings—neither "infallible gods" nor the "malevolent manipulators" (nor the stereotypic "eccentric buffoon," "evil-minded doctor," etc., that I mentioned earlier). Most do their job skillfully, and lead ordinary family and personal lives as well.
- Limit the "Freudian stereotype"—male therapist with a beard, a German accent, a pipe, and a detached manner—to historically accurate portrayals.
- Show working with severely mentally ill individuals as a specialty—most psychiatrists and psychologists don't regularly treat severe mental illnesses like schizophrenia or manic-depression.
- Include mental health professionals as supporting characters in stories having nothing to do with mental illness.

Depicting Treatment Facilities and Services for Those with Mental Illness

- Include depictions of effective treatments for mental illnesses other than psychotherapy, e.g., medications that can effectively treat depression and schizophrenia.

> • Show community facilities such as halfway houses, group homes, and day treatment centers as alternatives to traditional "mental hospitals."
> • Show that carefully coordinated teams of professionals now treat those with mental illnesses.
> • Have characters make statements about the benefits of treatments—for instance, "I got treatment and it helped."

When the radio personalities in Rome, Georgia, made jokes about the patients in the nearby psychiatric hospital, a group of people from the media and from the county's Mental Health Association got together and started talking about stigma and how destructive it was. The result was a media resolution signed by all the local television and radio stations. It reads: "We the undersigned desire to contribute to eradicating the stigma of mental illness. We will not be turned from our mission until the stigma ceases to exist in the hearts and minds of those around us."

Similarly, a quick response from mental health advocates led to the swift removal from the air of the offending advertisements for the TV program *Frasier.* In addition, some local television stations and the syndicator, Paramount TV, apologized and offered to show public service announcements to help educate the public about obsessive-compulsive disorders.

Perhaps one day, measures like these will no longer be necessary. Perhaps one day everyone will appreciate the true nature of mental illnesses and there will be no stigma. Perhaps one day compassion and not derision will be the natural response to mental illness. I look forward to that day.

Epilogue

Hope for the Future

W e are coming out of the Dark Ages in our understanding and treatment of those who suffer from mental illnesses. We have made great progress in changing attitudes. Less than twenty years after Thomas Eagleton was forced to drop out of the vice presidential race because of earlier treatment for a mental problem, Florida's former senator Lawton Chiles was elected governor of the state even after his disclosure that he had been taking Prozac. Chiles had suffered from depression following quadruple bypass heart surgery and had retired from the U.S. Senate because of "burnout." But he won the Democratic primary in 1990 with 69 percent of the vote and then ousted the Republican incumbent to become an active, hands-on governor. "I wish I'd known about Prozac [earlier]," Chiles said publicly, "because it helped me a lot."[1]

And we have new strength in Congress. Important consumer and family organizations such as the National Alliance for the Mentally Ill, the National Mental Health Association, and the Anxiety Disorders Association of America, among others, are stronger and more effective than ever. Most important, these national organizations have joined together to form a coalition that has positively influenced the debate over health care reform and insurance parity.

Small but important victories have also been achieved in the use of Social Security benefits and Medicaid to support people with severe mental illnesses in the community. The Fair Housing Act and the Americans with Disabilities Act now prevent discrimination against people who have mental disorders. Slowly, those with mental or emotional problems are being specifically included in programs designed to protect and support them.

We have learned much about how to influence the media, to change public attitudes, and shape public policy. But we have learned even more about the brain and how to treat many mental illnesses more effectively. In *An Unquiet Mind,* Kay Redfield Jamison captures the fervent scientific activity when she writes "There is a wonderful kind of excitement in modern neuroscience, a romantic, moon-walk sense of exploring and setting out for new frontiers . . . the pace of discovery [is] absolutely staggering."[2]

Every day I gather more evidence of the impact that these discoveries and the dedication of thousands of clinical professionals around the nation are having on individuals struggling to overcome their conditions. I have received letters from countless citizens. Many share their tales of sorrow, but much like Kathy Cronkite, Jerilyn Ross, Stuart Perry, and Angela Koppenol, others tell of optimism, of newfound health, and of lost lives regained. They offer us hope:

• "About five months ago, I finally got help for my depression. I was so depressed, I tried to kill myself. But the doctors and nurses at the hospital saved my life. They sent me to a psychiatrist who helped me get my life back. Even my family doctor couldn't believe the change in me. He told me he could see I have better control of my life now. I have done a 180-degree turnaround."

• "Over the years, I've watched my friend with OCD fight his illness and, with his unique combination of faith and strength, he has valiantly soared at times from the deepest despair and has made contributions to society."

• "This program has made the difference for my nephew between being a boy headed for jail and a wonderful young man now in college. I volunteer at the program because there is never enough that I can do to repay what they have done for our family."

• "We have found a psychiatrist who understands my wife and has her on medication that lets her lead a normal life."

• "I got in touch with Vocational Rehabilitation. They paid for me to continue in therapy and for my gas and prescriptions for a year until I could get on my feet. I was lucky. I stayed in intensive therapy. I eventually went to graduate school and got a degree in nursing. . . . I went on to become a psychiatric nurse, working with people just like me."

• "I began behavior modification therapy and it turned my life around. It enabled me to be self-supporting and live a normal life, for which I am grateful."

• "My doctor is the reason for my recovery from agoraphobia. I was a prisoner of my apartment for twenty-three years. I have been helped in taking baby steps out of such a critical illness. I was devastated and traumatized for these twenty-three years, until I finally was cared for by my doctor. I have been in daily group sessions and observed by my doctors on a daily basis. Gradually I have been weaned from my apartment. Today, my mind is being restored to a normal functioning capacity."

• "A wonderful physician and a caring caseworker have helped my son so much that he is now balanced out in his medication. He is going to a mental health program in our county and doing well. . . . His wonderful caseworker tells him he has great potential and is helping him immensely. . . . He hopes now to go to school to become a counselor himself."

• "I continue to take my medication and hope to get a degree in English literature. . . . Life is a wonderful thing and can be rewarding. I almost lost my life when I attempted suicide a decade ago, but new life is like clay to be molded into a fine sculpture."

Even the current generation of psychiatric "wonder drugs" may pale in comparison to what is to come. Within the next five years, scientists are predicting that we will have faster-acting, more effective medications with fewer side effects, drugs that are targeted more specifically to particular neurotransmitters and their receptors. Some researchers even speculate that in a decade or two, there will be medications that prevent mental illnesses from developing in the first place in people who are genetically vulnerable.[3]

Important progress has also been made toward the prevention of some forms of mental disorders. We have learned much about biological risk factors and even more about psychological and social risk factors. And there are now many programs across the country implementing prevention strategies to protect those at risk and to significantly enhance the possibilities of both physical and mental well-being. Beverly Long, who participated in both the President's Commission in 1978 and the Institute of Medicine's 1994 prevention study, has reminded me that the world of prevention today is vastly different from what it was two decades ago. "An assessment of the current scientific research and credible knowledge related to mental, neurological, and behavioral disorders clearly documents the tremendous advances," she told me recently.

Jimmy's mother, Miss Lillian, was a great baseball fan. She often quoted Yogi Berra of baseball fame, who is reputed to have said "The future ain't what it used to be." In thinking about the future for those with mental illnesses, what could be more apt? The bright future that lies before us was unimaginable when I first became involved in mental health in 1971.

The Tasks Ahead

While it is true that much progress has been made, there is still much to be done before the problems we face can be resolved. Our major challenges include:

Access to Treatment

Many who could benefit from treatment are still not receiving it. Even those with the most severe and persistent mental illnesses could improve with the new medications and rehabilitation, yet the hope of recovery is denied to hundreds of thousands because of a lack of access to care.

Many who could benefit remain incapacitated because they can't pay or because they live in rural areas where no services are available. Hundreds of thousands who suffer, and their families, face serious economic hardship because of limited insurance coverage under most existing plans. I receive so many letters from distraught family members, describing their heavy financial burdens and their frustrated efforts in trying to care for mentally ill loved ones. The stark reality is that our current system of public and private insurance discriminates badly against those in need of a broad array of mental health services.

Scientific Advances

On the scientific front, the biological basis of mental illnesses, most notably schizophrenia, has not yet yielded up all its secrets.

David Pickar[4] at NIMH told me during our recent meeting there, "We are one third of the way to where we want to be, especially with the treatment of schizophrenia. We have not yet hit the golden age—but we are getting closer." It is my deepest hope that this day will come soon.

Focusing on Children's Mental Health

Children's mental health and early intervention still have not gotten enough attention. Ever since the first White House Conference on Children in 1909, there have been meetings and conferences and commissions, all of which have told the same story—children with emotional problems don't receive the help they need. There have been recommendations on how to meet their needs and some progress has been made, but the agenda is far from finished.

Why, despite our long-term common understanding of the problems of children, have we failed to act decisively and powerfully to provide the best possible care for them? Few on either side of the political or ideological spectrum would argue that our children are not at risk. Few would disagree that there is a general breakdown in family structures; that poverty, abuse, neglect, violence, fear, hate, anger, and a hundred other problems threaten our children, our families, and clearly the future of our country.

So why is there such apathy about protecting our children from the moral, mental, and physical threats that are so obvious? Why isn't there more of a national recognition of the needs of children? Why isn't there more of an outcry to provide them with a greater sense of security, health, and hope?

At our tenth annual mental health symposium at The Carter Center, we focused on children and families at risk. There was a broad-based consensus among participants that, in its failure to act for our children's future, our country is depleting its clearest vision, its most important resource, its most fragile and most promising hope for tomorrow.

Changes are under way in mental health care and child welfare, income supports, health care, education, employment, and training. Government is being redesigned. And, while Congress has taken steps to extend health insurance coverage to an estimated 2.5 million uninsured and working poor children (and that is a positive development), there is still so much more that needs to be done to address the outcomes we would like to see for children and their families.

Perhaps it is that we do not have a clear focus, perhaps we lack a coordinated strategy, or perhaps there is a lack of political will to pursue the issue. Perhaps it is because our society has difficulty thinking about the future over the long term. Unfortunately, there are no quick solutions to the problems that plague us most.

We need a clear vision, drawing from our collective ideas and strategies, that will help create a national movement for children. We need to invest in research that will help us minimize the risk factors and strengthen the protective conditions in communities across the nation.

Alliances across agencies, groups, families, schools, individuals, hospitals, and community institutions are the best ways to develop protective strategies.[5] More and more states are now experimenting with cross-agency collaboration because they have seen that the failure to do so is too costly in terms of both money and wasted lives. Indeed, it is time that we develop the same kind of systematic, epidemiological approach to mental illness prevention and health promotion that has been so successful in the field of public health. It's time that we make a concerted effort to bring together and integrate what is now a fractured, piecemeal system.

In the year 2009, we will witness the one hundredth anniversary of the first White House conference on the needs of America's children. Let's really have something to celebrate, but let's not wait until the year 2009. Our future and the lives of our children depend on it.

Focusing on Worldwide Mental Health

These days, no health issue is truly local or national, even though it may occur within a limited geographic area. All are ultimately global because our world is becoming so interrelated. Beyond our national boundaries, mental illness is also of grave concern. A 1995 Harvard report about the world's poorest people tells us that "while basic physical health has improved worldwide, mental health has remained stagnant or has deteriorated."[6]

Internationally, nearly 500 million people suffer from some type of mental illness, ranging from mild depression to chronic schizophrenia to substance abuse. Comprising half of the ten leading causes of disability, these illnesses account for 11 percent of incapacity in the world.

Numbers alone, however, do not reflect the suffering, frustration, and humiliation many people must bear because society fails to deal effectively—and compassionately—with mental health issues. Sadly, in some nations, it is still common for mentally ill persons to be shunned to the point of near isolation. We cannot afford to ignore such pain.

The World Federation for Mental Health, a nongovernmental association of mental health professionals and volunteers, has as its major goal the increase of knowledge and understanding in countries around the world about the importance of mental health in our lives and the human and financial devastation caused by mental disorders.

Today, I chair the World Federation's International Committee of Women Leaders for Mental Health. Established in 1992, the committee consists of more than forty members—royalty, heads of state, and first ladies—and provides them with an opportunity to promote mental health issues and devote more resources to addressing them.

In September of 1996, The Carter Center and the World Federation convened a meeting in Washington, D.C., of first ladies, ministers of health, and health experts from Latin America. Eight first ladies attended and twenty-five countries were represented. The discussion centered around how these leaders could use their positions in public life to focus attention on mental health. They all agreed to take on the subject as a personal issue in their countries, in part because women and children suffer disproportionately from indirect yet tragic links to mental illness: lack of education and health care, poverty, domestic violence, war. We are following up with them and assisting them in their efforts.

We held a similar meeting in Finland in the summer of 1997 with women leaders from Europe. Many of those who attended were first ladies from the countries of the former Soviet Union, and all participated actively in the program, describing conditions in their countries. Again we focused on the impact of mental health on families. It was an interesting and fruitful meeting.

We cannot afford to ignore the pain that mental illnesses bring to people worldwide. The commitment of this group of women leaders can be a model for others of influence and prestige to emulate in an effort to promote awareness of mental health issues in the world and improve the lives of those who suffer. Mental health must be placed on the international agenda.

What We Can Do

Today we are at a crossroads. We are faced with the opportunity to bring mental health into the mainstream of our concerns, and we cannot afford to fail. There are three key principles that must guide all of our activities:

First, we must end all discrimination against those with mental disorders. Discrimination has denied many the access to desperately needed services for far too long—and it continues to limit the resources available to pay for care.

Despite all the work that has been done and the progress we have made, the stigma of mental illness is still all too pervasive in our society. We need more prominent people like Patty Duke, William Styron, Mike Wallace, Art Buchwald, Willard Scott, Margot Kidder, Rodney Dangerfield, Dick Cavett, Kathy Cronkite, Kay Jamison, and Rod Steiger speaking out about their mental illnesses and about their treatment and recovery.

Kindness, empathy, and understanding must replace stigma in our hearts and minds. This means rethinking our own attitudes. It means raising our children so that if they are confronted with a mental illness in themselves, their families, or friends and neighbors, they aren't afraid or ashamed to seek help. It means speaking out on behalf of mentally ill people and working for their rights as citizens.

Secondly, we must recognize that to be healthy, one has to be mentally healthy. Mental health is an integral part of every person's health. Awareness of mental health problems needs to permeate the health care system. Primary care physicians, nurses, and physician assistants must all have sufficient knowledge about mental health and the interdependence between mind and body to know when intervention is necessary and who is best able to intervene.

Not many people outside the mental health field understand mental disorders or how treatable they are. Not only those in medicine, but policy makers, other health care providers, and the general public need to know more about advances in treatment. Those in the mental health field have a responsibility to bridge the gap.

Finally, we must recognize the need to direct our resources in new ways. Appropriate mental health care doesn't cost too much—but a lack of proper care has great emotional and financial consequences. Investing in early intervention, treatment, and follow-up care will prevent far more costly disability and even death.

We must not waver in our support of people with the most persistent disabling mental illnesses. We must ensure that these individuals have the comprehensive, coordinated services they need in the community and the resources to obtain more intensive care in times of crisis. But we also cannot turn our backs on the millions of other Americans—young and old, rich and poor, of every race and ethnic origin—who, at some point in their lives, will need some kind of treatment.

You and I know these people. They are our friends, neighbors, our colleagues at work; they are members of our families, ourselves—the young girl in despair because her home and life were torn apart by a hurricane; the depressed fifty-year-old father of two who lost his job and can't find work; the mother suddenly too frightened to leave her apartment.

Making change is not easy. It is a struggle against intolerance, ignorance, entrenched interests, and inertia. But we must always keep in mind what the struggle is about:

- Individual human dignity
- The recognition of the worth of every person, regardless of disability

- The right of people to enjoy equal opportunity and equal treatment in all aspects of life, including physical and mental health care
- The importance of reducing dependence for those who are suffering from mental and emotional problems
- The creation of new opportunities—through treatment and recovery—for individuals to become contributing members of their communities

Before she died, the great anthropologist Margaret Mead came to visit me at the White House. We talked of our shared interest in mental health. She said to me that if we select for our first consideration the most vulnerable among us—the emotionally disturbed child, the institutionalized person with psychosis, the street addict—then our whole culture is humanized. She believed that our value as individuals, our success as a society, could be measured by the compassion we show for the vulnerable. Can we measure up to Margaret Mead's standards?

Glossary of Scientific Terms

Addiction: A strong physiological or psychological dependence on a chemical substance. When the substance is removed, the individual experiences withdrawal symptoms. Narcotics, alcohol, and sedatives may produce addiction.

Agranulocytosis: A potentially life-threatening blood disorder that can suddenly reduce the number of infection-fighting white blood cells. It is a potential side effect of clozapine, a medication used to treat schizophrenia.

Amygdala: a small, almond-shaped region in the brain that recognizes and regulates emotions—especially fear and anger—and coordinates our response to danger.

Anafranil: See *clomipramine.*

Basal ganglia: A region in the brain that consists of two structures, the *caudate nucleus* and the *putamen,* which act as "automatic transmissions." The former moves thoughts along in the frontal cortex, or thinking part of the brain, and the latter moves thoughts along in the part of the brain that controls movement. In OCD, the caudate nucleus seems unable to shift the frontal cortex to the next thought, so the thought repeats endlessly.

Benzodiazepines: A class of anti-anxiety medications, like Xanax.

BuSpar: See *buspirone.*

Buspirone (BuSpar): A medication prescribed for anxiety that acts on serotonin. It is also used in the treatment of obsessive-compulsive disorder.

CAT (computerized axial tomography) scans: Imaging techniques that use computers to combine a series of X-rays to provide a clearer picture of the brain's structure than individual X-rays alone.

Caudate nucleus: The part of the basal ganglia responsible for moving thoughts along in the frontal cortex, or thinking part of the brain. It is the "gatekeeper" for the brain, helping us to decide which thoughts will be repeated. In obsessive-compulsive disorder, the caudate nucleus seems unable to shift the frontal cortex to the next thought, so the thought repeats endlessly.

Chlorpromazine: One of the best-known neuroleptics, prescribed since the early 1950s to treat schizophrenia. It is effective in quelling the hallucinations, delusions, and disorganized thinking ("positive symptoms") of schizophrenia. This drug is taken once a day and is relatively inexpensive. Chlorpromazine blocks D2 dopamine receptors.

Cingulate gyrus: A structure at the center of the brain that connects with our autonomic responses such as the fight-or-flight reaction when faced with danger. It may be responsible for the feelings of dread that surface when a person with obsessive-compulsive disorder is unable to wash his hands, check the doors, or otherwise fulfill his obsessions. In experimental situations in which OCD patients are given items that excite their fears (such as soiled towels), brain scans show that blood flow increases in this area as well as the caudate nucleus and the orbital cortex.

Clomipramine (Anafranil): A serotonin reuptake inhibitor (not selective) used as an antidepressant and for the treatment of obsessive-compulsive disorder.

Clozapine (Clozaril): A newer treatment for schizophrenia that is easier to tolerate than traditional neuroleptics such as Thorazine. Clozapine helps to ameliorate both the negative and the positive symptoms of schizophrenia and improves cognitive functioning such as the patient's ability to pay attention and remember. It may also reduce hostile, aggressive, and suicidal behavior. It can be sedating and has the potential serious side effect of agranulocytosis, a potentially life-threatening blood disorder, but may be used safely if the patient is monitored regularly.

Clozaril: See *clozapine*.

Cognitive-behavioral therapy: Developed by University of Pennsylvania psychologist Aaron T. Beck, this is a specific approach to dealing with depression. It is based on the theory that thoughts impact feelings and feelings impact thoughts.

Cortical subplate: A fetal brain structure meant to guide neurons to their final destinations. After achieving its task, it is preprogrammed to fade away.

Cortisol: A hormone that the body releases under stress.

Depakote: See *divalproex*.

Divalproex (Depakote): A new medication recently found to be effective in treating mania in bipolar disorder.

Dopamine: A trace neurotransmitter that regulates brain cell activity in regions of the brain critical to movement, cognition, and emotional states. Schizophrenia is linked to excessive amounts of this brain chemical. Parkinson's disease is linked to an insufficiency of dopamine.

Electroconvulsive therapy (ECT): A treatment for severe depression. The therapy involves a series of mild electrical currents administered to a sedated patient that affects the part of the brain that regulates mood and helps stimulate the production of precursors to serotonin and norepinephrine.

Fluoxetine (Prozac): The most widely prescribed antidepressant in the U.S. It is a selective serotonin reuptake inhibitor (SSRI). It produces fewer side effects than older antidepressant medications such as MAOIs and tricyclics.

Fluvoxamine (Luvox): An antidepressant that blocks the brain's reabsorption of serotonin, allowing more to circulate. Also approved for obsessive-compulsive disorder.

Frontal lobes of the cerebral cortex: The "gray matter" in the brain that is engaged in higher reasoning and cognition. This area constitutes nearly 30 percent of the brain and is linked to many other key brain structures. The frontal lobes integrate information coming from these other sources, helping us to place ideas in sequences, envision plans for the future, identify abstract concepts, and initiate behavior related to our goals.

Glutamate: A major brain chemical involved in 40 percent of all messages transmitted.

Hypomania: A phase in bipolar disorder that precedes a full-blown episode of mania. The individual may feel euphoric ("up," "alive," "creative," "productive") or irritable, but the state is less dramatic than mania and the individual is still in control.

Hypothalamus: A brain structure that regulates hormones and behaviors such as eating, drinking, and sexual activity.

Lithium: The most prescribed medication for bipolar or manic-depressive disorder. It stabilizes moods and prevents the recurrence of manic or depressive episodes by increasing serotonin levels and affecting norepinephrine and dopamine, among other chemicals.

Locus ceruleus: An area in the brain involved in the body's response to stressful situations. When unexpected events occur, it signals danger, and the neurons increase their activity, releasing norepinephrine. Norepinephrine produces feelings of anxiety, fear, and panic.

Luvox: See *fluvoxamine.*

Monoamine: The chemical the brain uses to reabsorb neurotransmitters like serotonin and norepinephrine.

Monoamine oxidase inhibitor antidepressants (MAOIs): Antidepressant medications such as Marplan, Nardil, and Parnate. These are thought to operate by retarding the breakdown of monoamines in the brain.

MRI (magnetic resonance imaging) scans: An imaging technique that detects molecular changes in the brain when it is exposed to a strong magnetic field. These scans can also identify structural brain abnormalities and changes in the volume of brain tissue.

Negative symptoms of schizophrenia: Emotional and social withdrawal, lack of motivation, reduced language and emotional expressiveness. These seriously impair personal relationships.

Neuroleptics: Medications developed in the 1950s to treat psychosis and schizophrenia. They have been effective in quelling the hallucinations, delusions, and disorganized thinking of schizophrenia but have little effect on the emotional and social withdrawal of the illness. They can have disturbing side effects that include dry mouth, blurred vision, weight gain, tremors or stiffness, and tardive dyskinesia. Neuroleptics include medications such as Thorazine, Mellaril, Haldol, Moban, and Stelazine.

Neuroscience: The study of the brain in fields as diverse as anatomy, physics, physiology, biochemistry, electronics, psychology, psychiatry, computer engineering, neurology, genetics, pharmacology, and neurosurgery.

Neurotransmitter: A chemical that the nerve cells themselves release to communicate with one another.

Norepinephrine: A neurotransmitter that regulates alertness and arousal, and is implicated in depression. A deficiency of norepinephrine may contribute to the fatigue and depressed mood of the illness.

Olanzapine (Zyprexa): A recently introduced anti-schizophrenia medication that may affect more areas of the brain than either clozapine or risperidone while having fewer side effects.

Orbital cortex: A brain structure located just over the eyes, at the underside of the frontal cortex. It is the circuit that helps the brain to detect errors and tells us whether something is right or wrong. (When there is an error, it "fires" in long bursts.) It is believed that obsessive thoughts and impulses are generated here. The orbital cortex shows up as a "hot spot" in PET scans of OCD patients' brains, meaning it is inappropriately activated. This may be the key to explaining why affected patients constantly believe that their environment requires them to take some kind of corrective action.

Paranoia: Delusions arranged in an orderly sequence, often of persecution, in an otherwise relatively intact person.

PET (positron emission tomography) and SPECT (single-photon-emission computed tomography) scans: Imaging techniques that reveal brain activity while it is occurring by measuring the amount of blood flow or the utilization of glucose in a region in the brain (the more blood flowing or glucose consumed, the greater the activity in that area). PET scans can create images of brain chemistry at minute concentrations.

Phobia: An irrational fear such as a fear of heights, dogs, water, open spaces, closed spaces, etc.

Positive symptoms of schizophrenia: Readily visible symptoms of the illness such as hallucinations, delusions, and disorganized thinking.

Prefrontal cortex: A specific area of the frontal lobes just over the eyes. This brain structure organizes and prioritizes the flow of information through the cortex. It is the seat of what is called the "working memory"—our ability to hold newly acquired bits of information and relate them to what we already know. It allows us to understand spoken language as well as accomplish tasks in which we must remember visual images that are no longer in view. It is also an area thought to be important in organizing emotional responses to socially significant or provocative situations.

Prozac: See *fluoxetine.*

Psychosis: A mental state in which an individual has an impaired perception of reality. He or she may hallucinate, become incoherent and delusional, and may display bizarre behavior. Psychosis is a symptom of schizophrenia but may also occur with severe depression and bipolar disorder.

Putamen: Part of the basal ganglia thought responsible for moving thoughts along in the region of the brain that controls movement.

Receptors: The sites on a cell to which neurotransmitters attach themselves or "bind" (much like a key fits into a lock) in order to send their message and activate that cell. Mental illnesses may occur if receptors for specific neurotransmitters are malfunctioning or inadequate.

Risperdal: See *risperidone.*

Risperidone (Risperdal): Currently the most widely prescribed medication for schizophrenia. It targets the same dopamine receptors as clozapine and has the same effect on positive and negative symptoms without the danger of causing agranulocytosis. It is also nonsedating.

Selective serotonin reuptake inhibitors (SSRIs): Antidepressants such as Prozac and Zoloft that block the brain's reabsorption of serotonin, allowing more to circulate.

Serotonin: A neurotransmitter implicated in depression. A serotonin deficiency may underlie the sleep problems, irritability, anxiety, and suicidal behavior associated with depression.

Tardive dyskinesia: A sometimes irreversible condition that involves abnormal involuntary movements of the face, limbs, and, in some individuals, the whole body. A potential side effect of neuroleptic medications used in the treatment of schizophrenia.

Thalamus: The brain structure that helps us filter, process, and relay input from our senses, emotions, and memory.

Thorazine: See *chlorpromazine.*

Ventricles: The normally occurring spaces in the brain that act as reservoirs for cerebrospinal fluid. These spaces are enlarged in people with schizophrenia.

Zyprexa: See *olanzapine.*

Appendix A:
Other Common Mental Illnesses

Agoraphobia: Literally, fear of open spaces. An individual with this disorder is fearful of being in public places from which he or she perceives that escape may be difficult. Agoraphobia frequently accompanies panic disorder.

Alzheimer's disease: A disorder causing progressive, irreversible deterioration of brain function leading to impaired mental function and eventually death.

Antisocial personality disorder: A pattern of irresponsible behavior since the age of fifteen (see *conduct disorder*). Symptoms can include inability to sustain steady schooling or work (when work is available); failure to conform to social norms by performing acts that are subject to arrest (destroying property, harassing others, stealing); irritability and aggressiveness (assaults, child and spousal abuse); impulsiveness; lying; recklessness; child endangerment or neglect; inability to sustain relationships; lack of remorse.

Attention deficit hyperactivity disorder (ADHD): The most common of all childhood mental illnesses. Children with ADHD may fail at school, not because they lack intelligence, but because miswirings in the brain make it difficult for them to sit still and pay attention. They may talk out of turn and inappropriately, fidget restlessly, and suffer learning problems.

Autism: A lifelong condition that begins early and can disturb an individual's development. Once believed to be purely a psychological disorder—the result of faulty parenting—scientists now theorize that autism is primarily biological in origin. Recent studies have provided clear evidence of abnormalities in several regions of the brain related to this disorder.

Children with autism have difficulty establishing affectionate ties with their loved ones (no matter how caring their parents may be) and can respond in unusual or surprising ways to their environment. They may become rigid about rules, have difficulty processing information, overreact to normal daily events (or not react at all), suffer language deficits and speech impairments, and rock and babble to themselves for hours. About three quarters of children with autism are also mentally retarded.

Borderline personality disorder: Refers to a person who experiences unstable self-image and personal relationships with extreme mood swings and impulsivity. May result from a history of childhood sexual abuse or trauma.

Conduct disorder: A persistent pattern of behavior before age eighteen in which the rights of others and age-appropriate rules and norms are ignored. Symptoms can include stealing, running away, lying, fire-setting, truancy, breaking and entering, destruction of property, cruelty to animals, fighting, using a weapon, rape, cruelty to people. Almost half the children with conduct disorder become adults with antisocial traits.

Dysthymia: Chronic low-grade depression.

Eating disorders: Disturbances in eating behavior, including overeating, anorexia nervosa (self-starvation), and bulimia (bingeing and purging).

Hypochondria: An obsessive preoccupation with general health or a particular illness based on misinterpretation of body signals. It seems to mirror the fears and expectations of harm of those who suffer from obsessive-compulsive disorder.

Paranoid personality disorder: Refers to a person who is extremely distrustful, suspicious, and/or jealous of others, and frequently rigid and uncompromising. He or she can be highly critical of others and may interpret innocent remarks as personal attacks.

Personality disorders: Disorders in which individuals demonstrate personality traits that are inflexible and cause them either to adjust poorly in social relationships or to suffer internal distress. They include antisocial personality, borderline personality, and paranoid personality disorders.

Post-traumatic stress disorder (PTSD): An anxiety disorder occurring in the aftermath of a severe trauma: rape, assault, a serious accident, wartime experience, natural disaster, or other tragedy. People suffering from PTSD may constantly relive the trauma in nightmares or intrusive recurrent flashbacks, or they may withdraw into emotional numbness and depression. They may suddenly lash out in anger or isolate themselves from friends and family. PTSD can be associated with panic attacks and may lead its victims into substance abuse.

Schizoaffective disorder: A mental disorder characterized by symptoms of both schizophrenia and mood disorders such as depression or manic–depression.

Seasonal affective disorder (SAD): A form of depression. Sufferers become gloomy, oversleep, gain weight, and feel lethargic during fall and winter months.

Tourette's syndrome: A genetically determined neurological disorder characterized by intrusive thoughts and verbal and physical tics believed to result from dopamine/caudate nucleus dysfunction. Many people with Tourette's also suffer from obsessive-compulsive disorder.

Appendix B:
Frequency of Mental Illnesses Among Men and Women

Illness	Percentage of Men Affected	Percentage of Women Affected
Antisocial personality (manipulative exploitative, impulsive, aggressive)	5.8%	1.2%
Anxiety disorders	19.2%	30.5%
Attention deficit hyperactivity disorder (ADHD)	Estimates vary. Males three to nine times more likely to have ADHD	
Bipolar disorder (manic-depression)	1.6%	1.7%
Depression	12%	21.3% Women are twice as likely as men to be depressed
Schizophrenia	0.6% Early onset (age 15–45) more usual	0.8% Late onset (after age 45) more usual
Substance abuse	35.4%	17.9%

Based on Ronald C. Kessler, Katherine A. McGonagle, Shanyang Zhao, et al. "Lifetime and 12-Month Prevalence of DSM-III-R Psychiatric Disorders in the United States: Results from the National Co-Morbidity Survey," *Archives of General Psychiatry,* January 1994, and NIMH, *Women's Health Research Bulletin,* NIH publication no. 95-3827, Spring/Summer 1995.

Appendix C:
Side Effects of Antidepressants

As with all drugs, antidepressants occasionally cause side effects such as weight gain, skin rashes, dry mouth, palpitations, or stomach upset. Sometimes these side effects appear soon after treatment begins but weeks before the symptoms of depression dissipate. If severe, the side effects can interfere with a person's willingness to continue treatment. Many of these side effects do, however, disappear over time.

Appendix C

Likelihood of Experiencing Side Effects of Antidepressants

POTENTIAL SIDE EFFECTS

	Dry mouth Constipation Blurry vision	Drowsiness	Insomnia	Weight gain	Dizziness
Medications					
Cyclics					
Tofranil	moderate	low	low	moderate	moderate
Elavil	high	moderate	none	moderate	moderate
Newer cyclics (SSRIs)					
Prozac	none	none	moderate	none	none
Zoloft	none	none	moderate	none	none
Paxil	none	none	moderate	none	none
Monoamine oxidase inhibitors (MAOIs)					
Nardil	low	low	low	high	high
Parnate	none	none	moderate	none	high

The medications listed in this chart reflect only those discussed in this book. Because an individual's response to medication is unique, it is always best to consult with a psychiatrist or psychopharmacologist. Adapted from Mitch Golant and Susan K. Golant, *What to Do When Someone You Love Is Depressed* (New York: Villard Books, 1996).

Appendix D:
Resources You May Find Helpful

Books

GENERAL

Alliance for the Mentally Ill. *Mental Illness: A Handbook for Families.* Quebec, Canada: Alliance for the Mentally Ill, 1992.

Baron-Faust, Rita. *Mental Wellness for Women.* New York: William Morrow & Co., 1997.

Carter, Rosalynn, with Susan K. Golant. *Helping Yourself Help Others: A Book for Caregivers.* New York: Times Books, 1996.

Dowling, Collette. *You Mean I Don't Have to Feel This Way? New Help for Depression, Anxiety, and Addiction.* New York: Bantam Books, 1993.

Esser, Aristide H., and Sylvia D. Lacey. *Mental Illness: A Homecare Guide.* New York: John Wiley & Sons, 1989.

Fink, Jay Paul, and Allan Tasman. *Stigma and Mental Illness.* Washington, D.C.: American Psychiatric Press, 1992.

Frankl, Viktor. *Man's Search for Meaning.* New York: Pocket Books, 1988.

Goleman, Daniel. *Emotional Intelligence.* New York: Bantam Books, 1995.

Hales, Dianne, and Robert E. Hales. *Caring for the Mind: The Comprehensive Guide to Mental Health.* New York: Bantam Books, 1995.

Hamburg, David. *Today's Children: Creating a Future for a Generation in Crisis.* New York: Random House, 1992.

Hatfield, Agnes B. *Coping with Mental Illness in the Family: A Family Guide.* Arlington, Va.: National Alliance for the Mentally Ill, 1992.

Herman, Judith Lewis. *Trauma and Recovery.* New York: Basic Books, 1992.

Kass, Fredrick I., John M. Oldham, and Herbert Pardes, eds. *The Columbia University College of Physicians and Surgeons Complete Home Guide to Mental Health.* New York: Henry Holt & Co., 1992.

Koplewicz, Harold S., M.D. *It's Nobody's Fault: New Hope and Help for Difficult Children.* New York: Times Books, 1996.

Laskin, P., and A. Moskowitz. *Wish upon a Star: A Story for Children with a Parent Who Is Mentally Ill.* New York: Brunner/Mazel, 1991.

Lavin, Don, and Andrea Everett. *Working on the Dream: A Guide to Career Planning and Job Success.* Spring Lake Park, Minn.: Rise, Inc., 1996.

McElroy, Evelyn, ed. *Children and Adolescents with Mental Illness: A Parents' Guide.* Rockville, Md.: Woodbine House, 1988.

Pipher, Mary. *Reviving Ophelia: Saving the Selves of Adolescent Girls.* New York: Ballantine Books, 1994.

Pollin, Irene, with Susan K. Golant. *Taking Charge: How to Master the Eight Most Common Fears of Long-Term Illness.* New York: Times Books, 1996.

Shapiro, Joseph P. *No Pity: People with Disabilities Forging a New Civil Rights Movement.* New York: Times Books, 1994.

Swedo, Susan E., and Henrietta Leonard. *It's Not All in Your Head: The Real Causes and the Newest Solutions to Women's Most Common Health Problems.* San Francisco: HarperSanFrancisco, 1996.

Torrey, E. F. *Hidden Victims: An Eight Stage Healing Process for Families and Friends of the Mentally Ill.* New York: Doubleday, 1988.

Yudofsky, Stuart C., and Tom Furguson. *What You Need to Know About Psychiatric Medications.* New York: Ballantine Books, 1992.

SPECIFIC MENTAL ILLNESSES

Anxiety Disorders

Baer, Lee. *Getting Control: Overcoming Your Obsessions and Compulsions.* New York: Plume Books, 1992.

De Silva, W. P., and Stanley Rachman, eds. *Obsessive-Compulsive Disorder: The Facts.* New York: Oxford University Press, 1995.

De Silva, W. P., and Stanley Rachman, eds. *Panic Disorder: The Facts.* New York: Oxford University Press, 1996.

Dowling, Collette. *You Mean I Don't Have to Feel This Way? New Help for Depression, Anxiety, and Addiction.* New York: Bantam Books, 1993.

Dumont, Raeanne. *The Sky Is Falling: Understanding and Coping with Phobias, Panic, and Obsessive-Compulsive Disorder.* New York: W. W. Norton, 1996.

Levenkron, Steven. *Obsessive Compulsive Disorders: Treating and Understanding Crippling Habits.* New York: Warner Books, 1992.

Neziroglu, Fugen A., and Jose A. Yaryura-Tobias. *Over and Over Again: Understanding Obsessive-Compulsive Disorder.* San Francisco: Jossey-Bass, 1997.

Rapoport, Judith. *The Boy Who Couldn't Stop Washing: The Experience and Treatment of Obsessive-Compulsive Disorder.* New York: NAL-Dutton, 1990.

Ross, Jerilyn. *Triumph over Fear: A Book of Help and Hope for People with Anxiety, Panic Attacks, and Phobias.* New York: Bantam Books, 1994.

Schwartz, Jeffrey M. *Brain Lock: Free Yourself from Obsessive-Compulsive Behavior.* New York: HarperCollins, 1996.

Steketee, Gail S. *Treatment of Obsessive Compulsive Disorder.* New York: Guilford Press, 1996.

Zuercher-White, Elke. *An End to Panic: Breakthrough Techniques for Overcoming Panic Disorder.* Oakland, Calif.: New Harbinger Publications, 1995.

Bipolar Disorder

Berger, Diane, and Lisa Berger. *We Heard the Angels of Madness: A Family Guide to Coping with Manic Depression.* Quill, 1992.

Copeland, Mary Ellen. *Living Without Depression and Manic Depression: A Workbook for Maintaining Mood Stability.* Oakland, Calif.: New Harbinger Publications, 1994.

Duke, Patty, and Gloria Hochman. *A Brilliant Madness: Living with Manic Depressive Illness.* New York: Bantam Books, 1993.

Goodwin, Fredrick K., and Kay Redfield Jamison. *Manic Depressive Illness.* New York: Oxford University Press, 1990.

Jamison, Kay Redfield. *An Unquiet Mind: A Memoir of Moods and Madness.* New York: Knopf, 1995.

Torrey, E. Fuller, Ann E. Bowler, Edward H. Taylor, et al. *Schizophrenia and Manic Depressive Disorder: The Biological Roots of Mental Illness as Revealed by the Landmark Study of Identical Twins.* New York: Basic Books, 1995.

Whybrow, Peter C. *A Mood Apart: Depression, Mania, and Other Afflictions of the Self.* New York: HarperCollins, 1997.

Depression

Appleton, William S. *Prozac and the New Antidepressants: What You Need to Know About Prozac, Zoloft, Paxil, Luvox, Wellbutrin, Effexor, Serzone, and More.* New York: Plume Books, 1997.

Beck, Aaron. *Love Is Never Enough.* New York: Harper & Row, 1988.

Burns, David D. *Feeling Good: The New Mood Therapy.* New York: Avon Books, 1992.

Copeland, Mary Ellen. *Living Without Depression and Manic Depression: A Workbook for Maintaining Mood Stability.* Oakland, Calif.: New Harbinger Publications, 1994.

Cronkite, Kathy. *On the Edge of Darkness.* New York: Delta Books, 1994.

Dowling, Collette. *You Mean I Don't Have to Feel This Way? New Help for Depression, Anxiety, and Addiction.* New York: Bantam Books, 1993.

Dukakis, Kitty. *Now You Know.* New York: Simon & Schuster, 1990.

Elfenbein, Debra. *Living with Prozac and Other Serotonin-Reuptake Inhibitors.* San Francisco: HarperSanFrancisco, 1995.

Golant, Mitch, and Susan K. Golant. *What to Do When Someone You Love Is Depressed.* New York: Villard Books, 1996.

Gold, Mark S., and Lois B. Morris. *The Good News About Depression.* New York: Bantam Books, 1995.

Greist, John H., and James W. Jefferson. *Depression and Its Treatment,* rev. ed. Washington, D.C.: American Psychiatric Press, 1992.

Heckler, Richard A. *Waking Up Alive: The Descent, the Suicide Attempt, and the Return to Life.* New York: Ballantine Books, 1994.

Jack, Dana Crowley. *Women and Depression.* New York: HarperCollins, 1991.

Klein, Donald F., and Paul H. Wender. *Understanding Depression: A Complete Guide to Its Diagnosis and Treatment.* New York: Oxford University Press, 1994.

Kleinman, Karen R., and Valerie Raskin. *This Isn't What I Expected: Overcoming Post-Partum Depression.* New York: Bantam Books, 1995.

Kramer, Peter D. *Listening to Prozac.* New York: Viking Penguin, 1993.

Oster, Gerald D., and Sarah S. Montgomery. *Helping Your Depressed Teenager: A Guide for Parents and Caregivers.* New York: John Wiley & Sons, 1995.

Papolos, Dimitri, and Janice Papolos. *Overcoming Depression,* 3d ed. New York: HarperCollins, 1997.

Podell, Ronald M., with Porter Shimer. *Contagious Emotions: Staying Well When Your Loved One is Depressed.* New York: Pocket Books, 1992.

Rosen, Laura Epstein, and Xavier F. Amador. *When Someone You Love Is Depressed.* New York: Free Press, 1996.

Rosenthal, Norman E. *Winter Blues: Seasonal Affective Disorder: What It Is and How to Overcome It.* New York: Guilford Press, 1993.

Seligman, Martin E. P. *Learned Optimism: How to Change Your Mind and Your Life.* New York: Pocket Books, 1990.

Somer, Elizabeth. *Food and Mood: The Complete Guide to Eating Well and Feeling Your Best.* New York: Henry Holt & Co., 1995.

Styron, William. *Darkness Visible: A Memoir of Madness.* New York: Random House, 1990.

Whybrow, Peter C. *A Mood Apart: Depression, Mania, and Other Afflictions of the Self.* New York: HarperCollins, 1997.

Wurtzel, Elizabeth. *Prozac Nation: Young and Depressed in America.* New York: Riverhead Books, 1995.

Yapko, Michael D. *Breaking the Patterns of Depression.* New York: Doubleday, 1997.

Schizophrenia

Backlar, Patricia. *The Family Face of Schizophrenia: True Stories of Mental Illness with Practical Advice from America's Leading Experts.* Los Angeles: J. P. Tarcher, 1995.

Degen, Kathleen, and Ellen Deborah Nasper. *Return from Madness: Psychotherapy with People Taking the New Antipsychotic Medications and Emerging from Severe, Lifelong, and Disabling Schizophrenia.* Northvale, N.J.: Jason Aronson, 1996.

Deveson, Anne. *Tell Me I'm Here: One Family's Experience of Schizophrenia.* New York: Penguin, 1992.

Holley, Tara Elgin, and Joe Holley. *My Mother's Keeper: A Daughter's Memoir of Growing Up in the Shadow of Schizophrenia.* New York: William Morrow & Co., 1997.

Johnson, Angela. *Humming Whispers.* Point, 1996. (A young adult novel.)

Keefe, Richard S. E., and Philip D. Harvey. *Understanding Schizophrenia: A Guide to the New Research on Causes and Treatment.* New York: Free Press, 1994.

Moorman, Margaret. *My Sister's Keeper: Living with a Sibling's Schizophrenia.* New York: Viking Penguin, 1993.

Mueser, Kim T., and Susan Gingerich. *Coping with Schizophrenia: A Guide for Families.* Oakland, Calif.: New Harbinger Publications, 1994.

Siegel, Ronald K. *Whispers: The Voices of Paranoia.* New York: Crown, 1994.

Simon, Clea. *Mad House: Growing up in the Shadow of Mentally Ill Siblings.* New York: Doubleday, 1997.

Torrey, E. Fuller. *Surviving Schizophrenia: A Family Manual.* New York: Harper & Row, 1983.

Torrey, E. Fuller, Ann E. Bowler, Edward H. Taylor, et al. *Schizophrenia and Manic Depressive Disorder: The Biological Roots of Mental Illness as Revealed by the Landmark Study of Identical Twins.* New York: Basic Books, 1995.

OTHER ISSUES

Aging

Butler, Robert N., Myrna I. Lewis, and Trey Sutherland. *Aging and Mental Health,* 4th ed. New York: Merrill/Macmillan, 1991.

Attention Deficit Disorder

Barkely, Russell. *Attention Deficit Hyperactivity Disorder: A Handbook for Diagnosis and Treatment.* New York: Guilford Press, 1990.

Garber, Stephen W., Marianne Daniels Garber, and Robyn Freedman Spizman. *Beyond Ritalin.* New York: Villard Books, 1996.

Hallowell, Edward M., and John J. Ratey. *Driven to Distraction: Recognizing and Coping with Attention Deficit Disorder from Childhood Through Adulthood.* New York: Touchstone, 1995.

Autism

Grandin, Temple. *Thinking in Pictures, and Other Reports from My Life with Autism.* New York: Vintage, 1996.

Greenfield, Josh. *A Place for Noah.* New York: Pocket Books, 1979.

Harris, Sandra L. *Siblings of Children with Autism.* Rockville, Md.: Woodbine House, 1994.

Hart, Charles A. *A Parent's Guide to Autism.* New York: Pocket Books, 1993.

Williams, Donna. *Nobody Nowhere: The Extraordinary Autobiography of an Autistic.* New York: Avon Books, 1994.

Williams, Donna. *Like Color to the Blind.* New York: Times Books, 1996.

Disturbed Family Relations, Violence, and Post-Traumatic Stress Disorder

Allen, Jon G. *Coping with Trauma: A Guide to Self-Understanding.* Washington, D.C.: American Psychiatric Press, 1995.

Bass, Ellen, and Laura Davis. *The Courage to Heal: A Guide for Women Survivors of Child Sexual Abuse.* New York: HarperCollins, 1994.

Brooks, Barbara, and Paula M. Siegel. *The Scared Child: Helping Kids Overcome Traumatic Events.* New York: John Wiley & Sons, 1996.

DeBecker, Gavin. *The Gift of Fear: Survival Signs That Protect Us from Violence.* Boston: Little, Brown, 1997.

Dutton, Donald G., with Susan K. Golant. *The Batterer: A Psychological Profile.* New York: Basic Books, 1995.

Engel, Beverly. *The Emotionally Abused Woman: Overcoming Destructive Patterns and Reclaiming Yourself.* New York: Fawcett, 1992.

Engel, Beverly. *The Right to Innocence: Healing the Trauma of Childhood Sexual Abuse.* New York: Ivy Books, 1991.

Frankl, Viktor. *Man's Search for Meaning.* New York: Pocket Books, 1988.

Herman, Judith Lewis. *Trauma and Recovery.* New York: Basic Books, 1992.

Hybels-Steer, Mariann. *Aftermath: Survive and Overcome Trauma.* New York: Fireside, 1995.

Magid, Ken, and Carole A. McKelvey. *High Risk: Children Without a Conscience.* New York: Bantam Books, 1988.

Matsakis, Aphrodite. *I Can't Get over It: A Handbook for Trauma Survivors.* Oakland, Calif.: New Harbinger Publications, 1996.

Miller, Alice. *The Drama of the Gifted Child: The Search for the True Self.* New York: Basic Books, 1994.

Miller, Alice. *Thou Shalt Not Be Aware: Society's Betrayal of the Child.* New York: NAL-Dutton, 1991.

Walker, Lenore E. *The Battered Woman.* New York: HarperCollins, 1980.

Eating Disorders

Bruch, Hilda. *The Golden Cage: The Enigma of Anorexia Nervosa.* New York: Vintage, 1979.

Claude-Pierre, Peggy. *The Secret Language of Eating Disorders: The Revolutionary New Approach to Understanding and Curing Anorexia and Bulimia.* New York: Times Books, 1997.

Roth, Geneen. *When Food is Love.* New York: Plume Books, 1992.

Substance Abuse

Alcoholics Anonymous. *Twelve Steps and Twelve Traditions.* New York: Alcoholics Anonymous World Services, 1990.

Blum, Kenneth, and James E. Payne. *Alcohol and the Addictive Brain.* New York: Free Press, 1990.

Covington, Stephanie S. *A Woman's Way Through the Twelve Steps.* Center City, Minn.: Hazelden Foundation, 1994.

Dowling, Collette. *You Mean I Don't Have to Feel This Way? New Help for Depression, Anxiety, and Addiction.* New York: Bantam Books, 1993.

Evans, Katie, and J. Michael Sullivan. *Dual Diagnosis.* New York: Guilford Press, 1990.

Tourette's Syndrome

Bruun, Ruth Dowling, and Bertel Bruun. *A Mind of Its Own: Tourette's Syndrome: A Story and a Guide.* New York: Oxford University Press, 1994.

Haerle, Tracy, ed. *Children with Tourette's Syndrome: A Parent's Guide.* Rockville, Md.: Woodbine House, 1992.

World Wide Web Sites

*Compiled by Ed Francell, Georgia Alliance for the Mentally Ill, Education Committee.

American Academy of Child and Adolescent Psychiatry*
www.aacap.org/web/aacap

American Psychiatric Association*
www.psych.org

American Psychiatric Press*
www.appi.org

Americans with Disabilities Act*
www.Usdoj.gov/crt/ada/adahom1.htm

Center for Psychiatric Rehabilitation*
www.bu.ed.sarpsych

Center for the Study of Issues in Public Mental Health*
www.rfmh.org/csipmh

The Dana Alliance for Brain Initiatives
www.dana.org

Dartmouth/New Hampshire Psychiatric Research Center*
www.dartmouth.edu/dms/psyhrc

Department of Labor—America's Job Bank
www.AJB.dni.us/

Depression After Delivery
www.behavenet.com/dadinc

Depression FAQ (frequently asked
questions)
avocado.pc.helsinki.fi:81/128
.214.75.66/%7Ejanne/asdfaq

Florida Mental Health Institute★
www.fmhi.usf.edu

Health Care Financing
Administration★
www.hcfa.gov

Internet Depression Resource List
earth.execpc.com/%7Ecorbeau

Joint Commission on
Accreditation Healthcare
Organizations★
www.jcaho.org

Journal of the California Alliance
for the Mentally Ill★
www.mhsource.com/hy/journal
.htm

Knowledge Exchange Network,
Center for Mental Health
Services, Substance Abuse and
Mental Health Services
Administration
www.mentalhealth.org

Mental Health Infosource★
www.mhsource.com

Michigan Department of Mental
Health★
www.mdmh.state.mi.us/bh

National Alliance for the
Mentally Ill (NAMI)
www.cais.net/vikings/nami

National Alliance for the
Mentally Ill (NAMI)★
www.nami.org

National Association of State
Mental Health Program
Director's Institute★
www.nasmhpd.org

National Federation of Interfaith
Volunteer Caregivers, Inc.
www.NFIVC.org

National Foundation for Brain
Research
www.brainnet.org

National Institute of Child
Health and Human
Development
www.nih.gov/nichd

National Institute of Mental
Health
www.nimh.nih.gov

National Institute on Aging,
Alzheimer's Disease Education
and Referral Service
www.alzheimers.org

National Institute on Alcohol
Abuse and Alcoholism
www.niaaa.nih.gov

National Institute on Drug Abuse
www.nida.nih.gov

National Mental Health
Association★
www.nmha.gov

Ohio Department of Mental
Health★
www.mh.state.oh.us/system/
prime.html

Open Minds (managed care
consulting)★
www.openminds.com

Schizophrenia—Doctor's Guide
to the Internet★
www.pslgroup.com/shizophr
.htm

Texas Department of Mental
Health/Mental Retardation★
www.mhmr.state.tx.us/
mrmrco.htm

U.S. Department of Housing and
Urban Development★
www.hud.gov

U.S. Department of Veterans
Affairs★
www.va.gov

World Wide Web Mental Health
Home Page
www.mentalhealth.com

Organizations

INFORMATION CLEARINGHOUSES

ERIC Clearinghouse on Adult,
Career, and Vocational
Rehabilitation
The Ohio State University
2500 Kenny Road
Columbus, OH 43210-9983
(800) 848-4815

Knowledge Exchange Network
P.O. Box 42490
Washington, DC 20015
(800) 789-CMHS (2647)
(301) 443-9006

Electronic bulletin board:
(800) 790-CMHS (2647)

E-mail:
ken@mentalhealth.org

National Clearinghouse for
Alcohol and Drug Information
P.O. Box 2345
Rockville, MD 20847-2345
(301) 468-2600
(800) 729-6686

National Mental Health
Consumer's Self-Help
Clearinghouse
211 Chestnut Street, Suite 1000
Philadelphia, PA 19107
(215) 751-1810
(800) 553-4539

National Stigma Clearinghouse
275 Seventh Avenue, Lobby
Desk
New York, NY 10001
(212) 255-4411

GENERAL ORGANIZATIONS

American Academy of Child and
Adolescent Psychiatry
3615 Wisconsin Avenue, N.W.
Washington, DC 20016
(202) 966-7300

American Association for
Marriage and Family Therapy
1100 Seventeenth Street, N.W.
Tenth Floor
Washington, DC 20036
(202) 434-2277

American Association of Pastoral
Counselors
9504 A Lee Highway
Fairfax, VA 22031
(703) 385-6967

American Association of
Suicidology
2459 South Ash
Denver, CO 80222
(303) 692-0985

American College of Physicians
Department of Public
Education
Independence Mall West,
Sixth Street at Race
Philadelphia, PA 19106-1572
(800) 523-1546
(215) 351-2400 (in
Pennsylvania)

American Group Psychotherapy
Association
25 East Twenty-first Street,
Sixth Floor

New York, NY 10010
(212) 477-2677

American Medical Association
515 North State Street
Chicago, IL 60610
(312) 464-5000

American Psychiatric Association
1400 K Street, N.W.
Washington, DC 20005
(202) 682-6000

American Psychological
Association
750 First Street, N.E.
Washington, DC 20036
(202) 336-5500

American School Health
Association
7263 State Route 43
P.O. Box 708
Kent, OH 44240
(216) 678-1601

Association for the Advancement
of Behavioral Therapy
15 West Thirty-sixth Street
New York, NY 10018
(212) 279-2677

The Beck Institute for Cognitive
Therapy and Research
GSB Building
City Line and Belmont
Avenues, Suite 700
Bala-Cynwyd, PA 19004-1610
(610) 664-3020

Black Psychiatrists of America
2730 Adeline Street
Oakland, CA 94607
(510) 465-1800

The Center for Cognitive
Therapy
University of Pennsylvania
133 South Thirty-sixth Street,
Room 602
Philadelphia, PA 19104
(215) 898-4100

The Dana Alliance for Brain
Initiatives
745 Fifth Avenue, Suite 700
New York, NY 10151
(212) 223-4040

Erase the Stigma (ETS)
c/o The Mental Health
Association of San Diego
2047 El Cajon Boulevard
San Diego, CA 92104
(619) 543-0412

National Alliance for Caregiving
7201 Wisconsin Avenue,
Suite 620
Bethesda, MD 20814-4810
(301) 718-8444

National Alliance for the
Mentally Ill (NAMI)
200 North Glebe Road,
Suite 1015
Arlington, VA 22203
(703) 524-7600
(800) 950-NAMI

National Association for the
Advancement of Psychoanalysis
American Board for
Accreditation and
Certification, Inc.
80 Eighth Avenue, Suite 1210
New York, NY 10010
(212) 741-0515

National Association of Private
Psychiatric Health Systems
1319 F Street, N.W., Suite 1000
Washington, DC 20004
(202) 393-6700

National Association of Social
Workers
750 First Street, N.E., Suite 700
Washington, DC 20002-4241
(202) 336-8200

National Community Mental
Healthcare Council
12300 Twinbrook Parkway,
Suite 320
Rockville, MD 20852
(301) 984-6200

National Family Caregivers
Association
9621 East Bexhill Drive
Kensington, MD 20895-3104
(800) 896-3650
(301) 942-6430

National Federation of Interfaith
Volunteer Caregivers, Inc.
368 Broadway, Suite 103
Kingston, NY 12401
(914) 331-1358
(800) 350-7838

National Institute of Child Health
and Human Development
31 Center Drive, MSC 2425
Building 31, Room 2A32
Bethesda, MD 20892-2425
(301) 496-5133

National Institute of Mental
Health (NIMH)
Information, Resources,
and Inquiries Branch
5600 Fishers Lane,
Room 7C-02
Rockville, MD 20857
(301) 443-4513

National Mental Health
Association

1021 Prince Street
Alexandria, VA 22314-2971
(800) 969-NMHA

Recovery, Inc.
802 North Dearborn Street
Chicago, IL 60610
(312) 337-5661

Suicide Research Unit
National Institute of Mental
Health (NIMH)
5600 Fishers Lane,
Room 10C-26
Rockville, MD 20857
(301) 443-4513

ORGANIZATIONS FOR SPECIFIC ILLNESSES

Anxiety Disorders
Anxiety Disorders Association of
America
6000 Executive Boulevard,
Suite 513
Rockville, MD 20852
(301) 231-9350

National Anxiety Foundation
3135 Custer Drive
Lexington, KY 40517-4001

Obsessive Compulsive
Anonymous
P.O. Box 215
New Hyde Park, NY 11040
(516) 741-4901

Obsessive Compulsive Foundation
P.O. Box 70
Milford, CT 06460

(203) 874-3843 (twenty-four-
hour information line)
(203) 874-5669
www.iglou.com.fairlight/oca

Obsessive Compulsive
Information Center
Dean Foundation
8000 Excelsior Drive, Suite 302
Madison, WI 53717-1914
(608) 836-8070

Panic Disorder Education Program
National Institute of Mental
Health
5600 Fishers Lane,
Room 7C-02
Rockville, MD 20857
(800) 64-PANIC

Depression and Bipolar Disorder
Depression After Delivery
  P.O. Box 1282
  Morrisville, PA 19067
  (215) 295-3994
  (800) 944-4PPD

Depression and Related Affective
  Disorders Association
  Johns Hopkins Hospital
  Meyer 3-181
  600 North Wolfe Street
  Baltimore, MD 21287-7381
  (410) 955-4647

Foundation for Depression and
  Manic Depression
  24 East Eighty-first Street,
  Suite 2B
  New York, NY 10028
  (212) 772-3400

Lithium Information Center
  8000 Excelsior Drive,
  Suite 302
  Madison, WI 53717
  (608) 836-8070

National Alliance for Research on
  Schizophrenia and Depression
  60 Cutter Mill Road,
  Suite 200
  Great Neck, NY 11021
  (516) 829-0091

National Alliance for the
  Mentally Ill (NAMI)
  200 North Glebe Road,
  Suite 1015
  Arlington, VA 22203

(703) 524-7600
(800) 950-NAMI

National Depressive and Manic
  Depressive Association
  730 North Franklin,
  Suite 501
  Chicago, IL 60610
  (800) 82-NDMDA
  (312) 642-0049

National Institute of Mental
  Health (NIMH)
  Depression Awareness,
  Recognition and Treatment
  (D/ART) Program
  5600 Fishers Lane,
  Room 10-85
  Rockville, MD 20857
  (301) 443-4140

National Organization for
  Seasonal Affective Disorder
  P.O. Box 40133
  Washington, DC 20016

Postpartum Support
  International
  (805) 967-7636

Schizophrenia
National Alliance for Research
  on Schizophrenia and
  Depression
  60 Cutter Mill Road,
  Suite 200
  Great Neck, NY 11021
  (516) 829-0091

National Alliance for the
Mentally Ill (NAMI)
200 North Glebe Road,
Suite 1015
Arlington, VA 22203
(703) 524-7600
(800) 950-NAMI

Tardive Dyskinesia/Tardive
Dystonia
4244 University Way, N.E.
P.O. Box 45732
Seattle, WA 98145
(206) 522-3166

ORGANIZATIONS IN RELATED AREAS

Aging

Administration on Aging
330 Independence Avenue, S.W.
Washington, DC 20201
(202) 619-0724

American Association of Geriatric
Psychiatry
7910 Woodmont Avenue,
Seventh Floor
Bethesda, MD 20814
(301) 654-7850

American Association of Retired
Persons (AARP)
601 E Street, N.W.
Washington, DC 20049
(800) 424-2277

National Council on the Aging
409 Third Street, S.W.,
Suite 200
Washington, DC 20024
(202) 479-1200

National Geriatric Psychiatry
Alliance
1201 Connecticut Avenue,
Suite 300
Washington, DC 20036
(888) INFO-GPA

National Institute on Aging
Alzheimer's Disease Education
and Referral Service
P.O. Box 8250
Silver Spring, MD 20907-8250
(800) 438-4380

AIDS

AIDS Hotline
(800) 342-AIDS

The U.S. Department of Health
and Human Services
Public Health Services
Centers for Disease Control
(800) 368-1019

Alzheimer's Disease

Alzheimer's Disease and Related
Disorders Association
919 North Michigan Avenue,
Suite 1000
Chicago, IL 60611
(800) 272-3900

National Institute on Aging
Alzheimer's Disease Education
and Referral Center
P.O. Box 8250
Silver Spring, MD 20907-8250
(800) 438-4380

Attention Deficit Hyperactivity Disorder
Children and Adults with
  Attention Deficit Disorders
  (CHADD)
499 N.W. Seventieth Avenue,
Suite 101
Plantation, FL 33317
(800) 233-4050

Learning Disabilities Association
  of America
4156 Library Road
Pittsburgh, PA 15234
(412) 341-1515

Autism
Autism Society of America
  7910 Woodmont Ave.,
Suite 650
Bethesda, MD 20814
(301) 657-0881
(800) 3-AUTISM

National Autism Hotline
(304) 525-8014

Cancer
American Cancer Society
  1599 Clifton Road, N.E.
Atlanta, GA 30329
(800) 227-2345

The Wellness Community,
  National
10921 Reed Hartman Highway,
Suite 215
Cincinnati, OH 45242
(513) 794-1116

Child Abuse
Parents Anonymous, Inc.
  675 West Foothill Boulevard,
  Suite 220
Claremont, CA 91711
(909) 621-6184

National Child Abuse Hotline
  Childhelp USA
1345 El Centro Avenue
P.O. Box 630
Hollywood, CA 90028
(800) 4ACHILD (422-4453)
(800) 2ACHILD (222-4453)
(TDD)

National Committee to Prevent
  Child Abuse
322 Michigan Avenue,
Suite 1600
Chicago, IL 60604
(800) CHILDREN (244-5373)

National Council on Child Abuse
  and Family Violence
1155 Connecticut Avenue, N.W.,
Suite 400
Washington, DC 20036
(800) 222-2000

Survivors of Incest Anonymous
  P.O. Box 21817
Baltimore, MD 21222-6817
(301) 282-3400

Chronic Fatigue Syndrome/Epstein Barr
CFIDS Association
(800) 442-3437

National Chronic Fatigue
  Syndrome Association
(816) 931-4777

Diabetes
American Diabetes Association
  P.O. Box 25757
  1660 Duke Street
  Alexandria, VA 22314
  (800) 828-8293

Domestic Violence
Batterers Anonymous
  8485 Tamarind Avenue, Suite D
  Fontana, CA 92335
  (714) 355-1100

National Domestic Violence
  Hot Line
  (800) 799-SAFE (7233)
  (800) 787-3224

National Organization for Victim
  Assistance
  1757 Park Road, N.W.
  Washington, DC 20010
  (800) TRY-NOVA (879-6682)
  access.digex.net/~nova

National Victim Center
  2111 Wilson Boulevard,
  Suite 300
  Arlington, VA 22201
  (703) 276-2880
  www.nvc.org

Eating Disorders
American Anorexia/Bulimia
  Association (AABA)
  293 Central Park West,
  Suite 1R
  New York, NY 10024
  (212) 879-8351

Anorexia Nervosa and Related
  Eating Disorders, Inc.
  (ANRED)
  P.O. Box 5102
  Eugene, OR 97405
  (541) 344-1144

National Association of Anorexia
  Nervosa and Associated
  Disorders (ANAD)
  P.O. Box 7
  Highland Park, IL 60035
  (847) 831-3438

National Eating Disorders
  Organization (NEDO)
  6655 South Yale Avenue
  Tulsa, OK 74136
  (918) 481-4044

Overeaters Anonymous
  (310) 618-8835
  www.hiwaay.net/
  recovery

Heart Disease
Mended Hearts
  c/o American Heart
  Association
  7272 Greenville Avenue
  Dallas, TX 75231
  (214) 706-1442

Homelessness
National Coalition for the
  Homeless
  1621 K Street, N.W., Suite 1004
  Washington, DC 20009
  (202) 775-1322

Parkinson's Disease

National Parkinson's Foundation
  1501 N.W. Ninth Avenue
  Miami, FL 33136
  (800) 327-4545

Parkinson Support Groups of
  America
  11376 Cherry Hill Road,
  Suite 204
  Beltsville, MD 20705
  (301) 937-1545

Stroke

National Institute of Neurological
  Disorders and Stroke
  9000 Rockville Parkway,
  Building 31, Room 8A-16
  Bethesda, MD 20892
  (301) 496-5751

Stroke Connection of the
  American Heart Association
  7272 Greenville Avenue
  Dallas, TX 75231
  (800) 553-6321

Substance Abuse

Al-Anon, Alateen, and Adult
  Children of Alcoholics
  Al-Anon Family Group
  Headquarters
  (800) 344-2666
  www.solar.rtd.utk.edu/~al-anon

Alcoholics Anonymous World
  Services
  (212) 870-3400
  www.casti.com/aa

American Council for Drug
  Education

204 Monroe Street
Rockville, MD 20850
(301) 294-0600

American Methadone Treatment
  Association
  217 Broadway, Suite 304
  New York, NY 10007
  (212) 566-5555

Center for Substance Abuse
  Treatment
  National Drug Information
  Treatment and Referral Hotline
  (800) 662-HELP
  (800) 66AYUDA (Spanish)

Cocaine Anonymous World
  Services
  (310) 559-5833 (national
  referral service)
  (800) 347-8998 (for meeting
  locations)
  www.ca.org

Cocaine Hotline
  (800) COCAINE

National Center for Substance
  Abuse Prevention
  Workplace Helpline
  Department AL
  P.O. Box 1909
  Rockville, MD 20852
  (800) 843-4971
  (800) WORKPLACE

National Council on Alcoholism
  and Drug Dependence
  12 West Twenty-first Street
  New York, NY 10010
  (800) NCA-CALL

National Institute on Alcohol
Abuse and Alcoholism
Office of Scientific
Communication
6000 Executive Boulevard,
Suite 409
Rockville, MD 20892-7003
(301) 443-3860

National Institute on Drug Abuse
5600 Fishers Lane, Room 10-05

Rockville, MD 20857
(301) 443-6480

Tourette's Syndrome
Tourette Syndrome Association
42-40 Bell Boulevard
Bayside, NY 11361-2820
(800) 237-0717
(718) 224-2999 (in New York)

EMPLOYMENT ISSUES AND RESOURCES

Center for Psychiatric
Rehabilitation
Boston University
730 Commonwealth Avenue
Boston, MA 02215
(617) 353-3549
(617) 353-7701 (TDD)

Department of Justice
Office of Americans with
Disabilities Act
Civil Rights Division
P.O. Box 66118
Washington, DC 20035
(202) 514-0301

Equal Employment Opportunity
Commission
1801 L Street, N.W.
Washington, DC 20507
(202) 663-4900
(800) 800-3302

Fountain House
425 West Forty-seventh Street
New York, NY 10036-2304
(212) 582-0340

Job Accommodation Network
West Virginia University
P.O. Box 6080
Morgantown, WV 26506
(800) 526-7234

Matrix Research Institute/
Penn Research and Training
Center on Mental Illness
and Work
6008 Wayne Avenue
Philadelphia, PA 19144
(215) 438-8200
(215) 438-1506 (TDD)

National Empowerment Center
20 Ballard Road
Lawrence, MA 01843
(800) 769-3728

National Rehabilitation
Information Center
8455 Colesville Road,
Suite 935
Silver Spring, MD 20910
(800) 346-2742

National Research and Training
  Center on Psychiatric Disability
  and Peer Support
104 South Michigan Avenue,
Suite 900
Chicago, IL 60603
(312) 422-8180
(312) 422-0740

Rehabilitation Services
  Administration
U.S. Department of Education

Switzer Building, Room 3211
330 C Street, S.W.
Washington, DC 20202-2574
(202) 205-5474
(for a free list of state vocational
rehabilitation agencies)

Rise, Inc.
8406 Sunset Road, N.E.
Spring Lake Park, MN 55432
(612) 786-8334

Notes

Part I Introduction

1. Cronkite, Kathy, *On the Edge of Darkness: Conversations About Conquering Depression* (New York: Delta Books, 1994), p. 17.

Chapter 1

1. NAMI family survey, *Family Perspectives on Meeting the Needs for Care of Severely Mentally Ill Relatives: A National Survey,* funded by the John D. and Catherine T. MacArthur Foundation, 1991.
   Johnstone, E. C., et al., "The Harrow (1975–1985) Study of the Disabilities and Circumstances of Schizophrenic Patients," British Journal of Psychiatry 159, suppl. 13 (1991).

Chapter 2

1. Mental Illnesses Awareness Guide MEDIA, American Psychiatric Association.

Chapter 3

1. McGrath, E., G. P. Keita, Bonnie Strickland, et al., *Women and Depression: Risk Factors and Treatment Issues* (Washington, D.C.: American Psychological Association, 1990).

2. Ibid.
3. Riger, Stephanie, and Pat Gilligan, "Women in Management: An Exploration of Competency Paradigms," *American Psychologist* 35 (1980): pp. 902–11.
4. Warrick, Pamela, "The Sad Truth About Men," *Los Angeles Times* (February 10, 1997), p. E1.
5. Rosen, Laura Epstein, and Xavier F. Amador, *When Someone You Love Is Depressed* (New York: Free Press, 1996), p. 165.
6. Comorbidity can refer to more than just the co-occurrence of a mental illness with substance abuse. In fact, a recent survey of more than eight thousand noninstitutionalized Americans between the ages of fifteen and fifty-four found that roughly one sixth of the general population struggles with *three or more* mental disorders. An individual could have, for example, depression, an anxiety disorder, and alcoholism. Kessler, Ronald C., Katherine A. McGonagle, et al., "Lifetime and 12-month Prevalence of DSM-III-R Psychiatric Disorders in the United States: Results from the National Comorbidity Study," *Archives of General Psychiatry* 51 (1994): pp. 8–19.
7. Styron, William, *Darkness Visible: A Memoir of Madness* (New York: Vintage Books, 1992), p. 43.
8. According to Alan I. Leshner, director of the National Institute on Drug Abuse, people with mental disorders are 2.7 times as likely to have a drug abuse disorder than the rest of the population, and those with substance abuse problems are 4.5 times as likely to have mental disorders. Leary, Warren E., "Depression Travels in Disguise with Other Illnesses," *The New York Times,* January 17, 1996.
9. Ibid.
10. Sleek, Scott, "When Depression Lurks Beneath an Addiction," *American Psychological Association Monitor,* January 1997, p. 33.
11. As described in a report to Congress by the Department of Health and Human Services: *National Plan for Research on Child and Adolescent Mental Disorders,* 1990. Also, between 17 and 22 percent of our children and adolescents—11 to 14 million young Americans—suffer from mental disorders that include the above illnesses as well as autism, Tourette's syndrome, and attention deficit hyperactivity disorder (ADHD).
12. Tanoye, Elyse, "Antidepressant Makers Study Kids' Market," *The Wall Street Journal,* April 4, 1997.

13. In 1994, about 2 million children were diagnosed with this disorder.

14. Sperling, Dan, "Families Struggle with Kids' Hyperactive Behavior," *USA Today,* February 6, 1990, p. 4D.

15. Larry B. Silver of Georgetown University School of Medicine in Washington, D.C.

16. Between 5 and 10 percent of all children suffer from anxiety disorders.

17. Frazier, Jean A., et al. "Brain Anatomic Magnetic Resonance Imaging in Childhood-Onset Schizophrenia." *Archives of General Psychiatry* 53 (1996): pp. 617–24.

18. In the U.S., white men over eighty are six times more likely to kill themselves than the rest of the population.

19. One third of the elderly who need mental health services receive it from mental health providers, one third from general health care providers who may not be as well versed in mental health issues, and one third receive no treatment at all.

20. Kolata, Gina, "Which Comes First: Depression or Heart Disease?" *The New York Times,* January 14, 1997.

21. Volz, Joe, "Depression Treatable Quickly and Effectively," *The Plain Dealer* (Cleveland), February 21, 1995, p. 10E.

22. Katz, Ira R., "Prevention of Suicide Through Education on Late Life Depression," testimony before the Senate Select Committee on Aging, Washington, D.C., July 30, 1996.

23. Bello, Kenya Napper, "Acute Depression is a Disease . . . Not a Character Flaw," *Black Men Don't Commit Suicide,* Spring 1995, p. 1.

24. Centers for Disease Control and Prevention, "*CDC Surveillance Summaries,*" *Morbidity and Mortality Weekly Report* 45, no. SS-4 (September 27, 1996).

25. National Coalition of Hispanic Health and Human Service Organizations, *Growing Up Hispanic.* Vol. II, *National Chartbook* (Washington, D.C.: National Coalition of Hispanic Health and Human Service Organizations, 1995).

26. First, Michael B., Allen Frances, and Harold Alan Pincus, *Diagnostic and Statistical Manual of Mental Disorders, DSM-IV™ Handbook of Differential Diagnosis* (Washington, D.C.: American Psychiatric Press, 1995).

27. Homeless people can have dental, gynecological, dermatological, heart, respiratory problems, and sexually transmitted diseases.

Homelessness also brings with it ailments caused by excessive exposure to heat and cold, malnutrition, and infectious diseases. Kass, Frederic, "Mental Illness and Homelessness," *Psychiatric News,* October 6, 1989, p. 3.

28. Those without addresses are difficult to count and definitions of homelessness vary.

29. A 1989 study in Baltimore of 528 homeless people living in missions and shelters found that 60 percent of the men and 70 percent of the women suffered from schizophrenia, a mood disorder, or an anxiety disorder. Breakey, William R., Pamela J. Fischer, M. Kramer, et al., "Health and Mental Health Problems of Homeless Men and Women in Baltimore," *Journal of the American Medical Association* 262 (1989): pp. 1352–57.

30. Rosenthal, A. M. "Park Avenue Lady" *The New York Times,* November 23, 1990.

Chapter 4

1. National Mental Health Association awareness campaign, "Understanding Mental Illness," 1992.

2. Swedo, Susan E., and Henrietta Leonard, *It's Not All in Your Head: The Real Causes and the Newest Solutions to Women's Most Common Health Problems* (San Francisco: HarperSanFrancisco, 1996).

3. Ibid.

4. This list is adapted from Baron-Faust, Rita, *Mental Wellness for Women* (New York: William Morrow & Co., 1997), pp. 252–53.

5. Gold, Mark S., and Lois B. Morris, *The Good News About Depression* (New York: Bantam Books, 1995), p. 238.

6. Perlmutter, Richard A., "A Clinical Family Approach to Anxiety Disorders," *ADAA Reporter,* Spring 1997, p. 2.

7. Produced in association with the Dana Alliance for Brain Initiatives, a nonprofit organization of 150 neuroscientists. *Grey Matters: A Conversation with Art Buchwald, William Styron, and Mike Wallace,* 1996 (audiotape).

8. *The GAMI News,* January/February 1997.

9. Gold, p. 268.

Chapter 5

1. Landers, Ann, "Mental Illness Is Often a Treatable Condition," *Los Angeles Times,* September 4, 1997, p. E3.
2. Pear, Robert, "Employers Told to Accommodate the Mentally Ill," *The New York Times,* April 30, 1997.
3. Kunde, Diana, "Employers Offer Help to Depressed Workers," *Sunday Oregonian,* March 12, 1995, p. B1.
4. Adapted from SAMHSA, *Mental Illness Is Not a Full-Time Job,* DHHS publication no. (SMA) 96-3102, U.S. Department of Health and Human Services, Substance Abuse and Mental Health Services Administration, 1996; and Lavin, Don, and Andrea Everett, *Working on the Dream: A Guide to Career Planning and Job Success* (Spring Lake Park, Minn.: Rise, Inc., 1996).
5. Karen Davis, president of the Commonwealth Fund, is a nationally recognized economist and an expert in public policy.
6. Umland, Beth, and Foster Higgins. "Foster Higgins National Survey: Trends and Behavioral Benefits." *Behavioral Healthcare Tomorrow,* June 1997, p. 58.
7. Miller, Andy, "Columbus Firms Champion Mental Health Coverage," *Mental Health Association of Georgia Messenger,* May 1997, p. 1.
8. Hymowitz, Carol, and Ellen Joan Pollock, "Psychobattle: Cost-Cutting Firms Monitor Couch Time as Therapists Fret," *The Wall Street Journal,* July 13, 1995, p. 1; Lewin, Tamar, "Questions of Privacy Roil Arena of Psychotherapy," *The New York Times,* May 22, 1996; and Moldawsky, Stanley, "Managed Care and Psychotherapy are Incompatible," *APA Monitor,* July 1997, p. 24.
9. Fox, Candace Smith, "The Most Powerful Family Intervention—The Letter," *Contra Costa AMI Newsletter,* November/December 1996.
10. Golant, Mitch, and Susan Golant, *What to Do When Someone You Love Is Depressed* (New York: Villard Books, 1996), pp. 89–91.
11. National Institute of Mental Health, *Schizophrenia: Questions and Answers, 1990,* DHHS publication no. (ADM) 86-1457, U.S. Department of Health and Human Services, National Institute of Mental Health, 1990.
12. Golant and Golant, p. 78.

13. Abraham, Dylan, "Getting Well Is Not a Race," *NAMI Advocate,* January/February 1997, p. 10.

Part II Introduction

1. Once the message is relayed, the neurotransmitters return to the nerve cell of origin or are broken down chemically.
2. Research has linked suicidal behavior, impulsiveness, aggression, and violence to reduced serotonin levels. Studies have associated high levels of serotonin with leadership. Addictions to substances such as cocaine and heroin are also related to drug-induced alterations in these neurotransmitters and their receptors.
3. Especially in treating individuals with anxiety disorders, obsessive-compulsive disorder, and depression.
4. Anthony, William A., "Changing Visions, Changing Lives: New Revolutions," *The CAMI Statement,* May/June, 1993, p. 1.
5. Ibid.

Chapter 6

1. While there is some natural variation in ventricle size among all of us, in studies of identical twins where one was afflicted and the other was not, it was found that the twin with schizophrenia had a larger ventricle area than the well twin. Because these enlarged spaces are present in young, recently diagnosed schizophrenia patients as well as older ones, scientists now believe that they have always been there and are not the result of the brain atrophying as a result of the disease or the side effects of medication.
2. Researchers have discovered abnormalities and asymmetries in other areas of the cortex. Some have located neurons that are turned inside out within the cortex. Others have found that some neurons have migrated to the wrong spot within the brain, leaving small regions permanently miswired or with faulty connections.
3. Schooler, Carmi, et al., "A Time Course Analysis of Stroop Interference and Facilitation: Comparing Normal Individuals and Individuals with Schizophrenia," *Journal of Experimental Psychology: General* 126 (March 1997).
4. According to Daniel Weinberger of the Clinical Brain Disorders Branch of NIMH, a fetal brain structure called the *cortical subplate*

is meant to guide neurons to their final destinations and then is preprogrammed to fade away. He speculates that perhaps a "pathological event" occurred during this crucial stage of development that might have interfered with this process and caused these various defects.

5. An epidemiological study of the consequences of a 1957 influenza epidemic in Finland, for example, found that individuals whose mothers were in the second trimester of pregnancy when they became ill had a significantly higher rate of hospitalization for schizophrenia than those whose mothers were exposed during a different trimester or not at all. More than a dozen other investigations back up this theory. Mednick, S. A., R. A. Machon, M. O. Huttunen, et al., "Adult Schizophrenia Following Prenatal Exposure to an Influenza Epidemic," *Archives of General Psychiatry* 45 (1988): pp. 189–92. Also Wyatt, Richard Jed, and Ioline D. Henter, "Schizophrenia: An Introduction," *Brain Work: The Neuroscience Newsletter*, May/June 1997, p. 3.

   Another study has linked an increased incidence of the illness in Dutch children to mothers who suffered severe starvation in early pregnancy during World War II. Weinberger, Daniel R., "From Neuropathology to Neurodevelopment," *The Lancet* 346 (1995): pp. 552–57.

6. Tyrone Cannon, a psychologist at the University of Pennsylvania, is studying the role of oxygen deprivation during gestation in the development of schizophrenia.

7. Hollister, J. Megginson, Peter Laing, and Sarnoff A. Mednick, "Rhesus Incompatibility as a Risk Factor for Schizophrenia in Male Adults," *Archives of General Psychiatry* 53 (1996): pp. 19–24.

8. A recent study at NIMH seems to confirm this theory. Using PET scans, Dr. Alan Breier and his colleagues have found a relationship between behavior and the amount of dopamine released in the brain. Those patients with the most psychotic symptoms showed the highest activation of dopamine.

   Scientists in Japan have also found that people with schizophrenia have an unusually low number of a particular dopamine receptor (called D1) in the prefrontal cortex. This is an area important for flexibility in planning and the control of impulses and emotions. D1 receptors have been shown to inhibit the action of D2 receptors, which are implicated in hallucinations. It is possible that D2 receptors could become overactive if there are not enough D1 receptors in force. Researchers in Sweden have found reduced D1 receptors in the basal ganglia, another key area of the brain, as well.

9. Dr. Kenneth S. Kendler and Dr. Scott R. Diehl of the Departments of Psychiatry and Genetics at Virginia Commonwealth University provide strong evidence that schizophrenia aggregates in families.

10. In 1992, there were seventy-six drugs in development for schizophrenia in the United States and forty-two more in other countries. PJB Publications, *Pharmacoprojects* (Surrey, England: PJB Publications, 1992).

    According to the Dana Alliance for Brain Initiatives, between 1995 and 1996, at least six new medications for the treatment of schizophrenia were undergoing human trials. The Dana Alliance for Brain Initiatives, *Brain Research for the Life of Your Mind: Progress and Promise* (Washington, D.C.: Dana Alliance, May 1996).

11. Risby, Emile, Deane Donnigan, and Charles Nemeroff, "Formulary Considerations for Treating Psychiatric Disorders: Schizophrenia," *Formulary* 23 (1997): pp. 142–55.

12. Up to 60 percent of patients who are resistant to neuroleptics do improve on clozapine when treated for a year. Sharma, Tonmoy, "Schizophrenia: Recent Advances in Psychopharmacology," *British Journal of Hospital Medicine* 55 (1996): pp. 194–98.

13. Clozapine improves the patient's ability to pay attention, remember, think straight, make choices, and exercise initiative. It may also reduce hostile, aggressive, and suicidal behavior, perhaps because it alleviates the feelings of depression and hopelessness. Ibid., p. 195.

14. Agranulocytosis, a potentially life-threatening blood disorder that can suddenly reduce the number of infection-fighting white blood cells. Clozapine can be used safely, with careful and regular monitoring.

15. Dr. Harriet Lefley, professor of psychiatry at the University of Miami, describes this case in "Awakenings and Recovery: Learning the Beat of a Different Drummer," *The Journal of the California Alliance of the Mentally Ill* 7 (July 1996): p. 4.

16. Risperidone can be prescribed to people who have just been diagnosed with schizophrenia (not only those who do not tolerate or

respond to neuroleptics), and it requires no weekly blood tests. It affords patients a great deal of freedom and mobility, and they seem to improve more and more over time. They even seem to gain better control over their abstract thought processes and their ability to follow directions. Raleigh, Fred, "A New Beginning," *The Journal of the California Alliance of the Mentally Ill* 7 (July 1996): pp. 7–9.

17. Mary D. Moller, a psychiatric nurse and administrator at the Suncrest Wellness Center in California, describes this case in "Learning from the Awakening," *The Journal of the California Alliance of the Mentally Ill* 7 (July 1996): p. 11.

18. Wingerson, Dane, "Awakenings—To What?" *The Journal of the California Alliance of the Mentally Ill* 7 (July 1996): p. 14.

19. Strauss, John S., "Pulling Themselves Together," *The Journal of the California Alliance of the Mentally Ill* 7 (July 1996): pp. 19–29.

20. Bellack, Alan S., and Kim T. Mueser, "Psychosocial Treatment for Schizophrenia," in *Special Report: Schizophrenia, 1993* (National Institute of Mental Health, 1993).

21. Wingerson, p. 14.

Chapter 7

1. However, the APA notes that "the disorder was three times more common among adopted children whose biological relatives suffered depression."

2. Leary, Warren E., "Depression Travels in Disguise with Other Illnesses," *The New York Times,* January 17, 1996.

3. Stress causes an overproduction of certain stress hormones such as *cortisol.* (Depressed individuals have been found to have an oversupply of cortisol and other stress hormones in their blood and spinal cord fluid.) Too much cortisol, in turn, may generate an imbalance in neurotransmitters.

4. Other neurotransmitters, especially norepinephrine. A decreased amount of norepinephrine, which regulates alertness and arousal, may contribute to the fatigue and depressed mood of the illness.

5. Neurons located in the frontal cortex.

6. Drevets, Wayne C., Joseph L. Price, Joseph R. Simpson, et al., "Subgenual Prefrontal Cortex Abnormalities in Mood Disorders," *Nature* 386 (1997): pp. 824–27.

7. The frontal cortex connects with other structures such as the amygdala that are thought to modulate the production of the neurotransmitters serotonin and norepinephrine. Dr. Wayne Drevets at the University of Pittsburgh has also found that the amygdala is overactive in people who are depressed—the greater the activity, the more profound the depression.

8. Dr. Mark S. Gold, professor of psychiatry at the University of Florida, in his book *The Good News About Depression*.

9. Dr. Norman E. Rosenthal, director of light therapy studies at the National Institute of Mental Health, in an interview reported in Kathy Cronkite's book *On the Edge of Darkness: Conversations About Conquering Depression*.

10. The sleep hormone is melatonin. Melatonin is a by-product of serotonin. The more melatonin in the system, the less serotonin. It is possible that an overabundance of melatonin (and a concomitant drop in serotonin levels) causes this type of depression.

11. Clinton D. Kilts, Ph.D., Department of Psychiatry, Emory University, Atlanta, Georgia, personal communication, 1996. Other researchers have used PET scans and electroencephalograms (EEGs) to predict who will respond to antidepressant medications.

12. Between 70 and 80 percent of depressed individuals respond to this kind of therapy. Imbalances in the neurotransmitters serotonin and norepinephrine are thought to underlie depression. Most antidepressants work by increasing these chemicals in the brain.

13. Scientists have wondered why it can take so long for the medication to become fully effective. It is now believed that one type of serotonin receptor acts as a damper, slowing the natural secretion of this neurotransmitter to keep it at a relatively fixed level in the brain, even as the medication helps to increase its concentration. It takes about three weeks for this brake to allow serotonin levels to rise. This can vary greatly from individual to individual. Older people, for example, metabolize these medications much more slowly, and therefore would require different doses than young adults. The search for the proper dosage for a given individual can also take some time.

14. Cyclic antidepressants block the absorption or *reuptake* of the neurotransmitters norepinephrine and serotonin. The older ones work mainly on norepinephrine, which acts in the brain to regu-

late anxiety and panic, while the newer ones block the body's re-absorption of serotonin, allowing for greater levels of it to circulate in the bloodstream. Prozac and other SSRIs have also been used to treat other mental illnesses such as eating disorders, hypochondria, and obsessive-compulsive disorder.

15. Internists and professors of psychiatry at the University of Wisconsin Medical School. Greist, John H., and James W. Jefferson, *Depression and Its Treatment,* rev. ed. (Washington, D.C.: American Psychiatric Press, 1992).

Chapter 8

1. He is also chief of the NIMH Clinical Neuroscience Branch.
2. According to the APA, close relatives of those suffering from the disorder are 10 to 20 times more likely to develop depression or manic-depression than the general public.
3. Drevets, Price, Simpson, et al., pp. 824–27. (Imaging studies of bipolar individuals are often limited to those who are in a depressed phase because it is difficult to scan patients who are experiencing manic symptoms.)
4. Landers, Ann, p. E3.
5. A recent NIMH report estimates that lithium treatment for manic-depressive illness has saved the U.S. economy more than $145 billion since 1970. U.S. Department of Health and Human Services, *Justification of Estimates for Appropriations Committees, Fiscal Year 1997,* Public Health Service, National Institutes of Health-Volume IV; National Institute of Mental Health, 1997, p. 15.

   It takes less than a week to alleviate symptoms. Although scientists have not yet determined exactly how it works, it is thought that lithium also impacts the neurotransmitters in the brain, increasing the serotonin levels and affecting norepinephrine and dopamine, among other chemicals. Lithium may also be prescribed to an individual who is suffering from depression, as an adjunct to other medications.
6. A professor of psychiatry at Johns Hopkins University.
7. Jamison, Kay Redfield, *An Unquiet Mind: A Memoir of Moods and Madness* (New York: Knopf, 1995), p. 118.
8. Ibid., pp. 127–28.

9. In preliminary findings presented by Dr. Gabor Keitner, a professor of psychiatry at Brown University, to the annual meeting of the American Psychiatric Association in 1997. Cited in "Family Therapy May Aid Recovery from Manic Depression," *The New York Times,* May 20, 1997.
10. Swedo and Leonard, p. 153.

Chapter 9

1. Klein, Rachel Gittleman, "Is Panic Disorder Associated with Childhood Separation Anxiety Disorder?" *Clinical Neuropharmacology* 18, suppl 2 (1995): pp. S7–S14.
2. Experiments with lab animals have suggested that under normal circumstances, certain neurons in the *locus ceruleus,* an area that is involved in the body's response to stressful situations, are programmed to recognize unexpected events. When they occur, it signals danger, and the neurons increase their activity, releasing norepinephrine. This neurotransmitter produces feelings of anxiety, fear, and panic.
3. According to Dr. Hans Breiter and his colleagues at Harvard University, including NIMH director Steven Hyman.
4. Ross, Jerilyn, *Triumph over Fear* (New York: Bantam Books, 1994), p. 78.
5. Ibid., p. 80.
6. Ibid., pp. 12–13.
7. Ibid., p. 23.
8. To date, more than a dozen different serotonin receptors have been identified in the brains of patients with OCD.
9. It is theorized that some deficit in certain serotonin receptors may heighten the stress response that those with OCD experience, producing a constant state of overarousal. Perhaps these abnormalities in brain chemistry are the result (or the cause) of the brain circuitry problems that have been identified in OCD patients.
10. The caudate nucleus. Tourette's syndrome, a disorder characterized by intrusive thoughts, verbal and physical tics, and OCD symptoms, is believed to result from the same dopamine/caudate nucleus dysfunction.
11. It has been theorized that abnormal serotonin levels might inhibit the activity of dopamine, which could lead to the fixed patterns

of obsessions and compulsions. Leonard, Henrietta L., Marge C. Lenane, and Susan E. Swedo, "Obsessive Compulsive Disorder," *Child and Adolescent Psychiatric Clinics of North America* 2 (1993): pp. 655–66.

12. The four areas are *basal ganglia, orbital cortex, cingulate gyrus, thalamus.* See the glossary for a detailed explanation of these structures.

13. Psychiatrist Jeffrey Schwartz in the OCD Research Group at UCLA's Neuropsychiatric Institute. Schwartz, Jeffrey M., *Brain Lock: Free Yourself from Obsessive-Compulsive Behavior* (New York: HarperCollins, 1996), p. 56.

14. The caudate nucleus, orbital cortex, cingulate gyrus, and thalamus.

15. Schwartz, p. xv.

Chapter 10

1. Albee, George, "Revolutions and Counterrevolutions in Prevention," *American Psychologist* 51 (1996): p. 1132.

2. National Advisory Mental Health Council, *National Plan for Research on Child and Adolescent Mental Disorders,* DHHS publication no. (ADM) 90-1683, U.S. Department of Health and Human Services, Alcohol, Drug Abuse, and Mental Health Administration, 1990, p. 22.

3. Azar, Beth, "Environment Is Key to Serotonin Levels," *American Psychological Association Monitor,* April 1997.

4. Reiss, David, *The Prevention of Mental Disorders: A National Research Agenda,* a report from the National Institute of Mental Health, 1994, quoted in "MH Coalition Highlights Value of Prevention, Research, Training," *Psychiatric News,* January 7, 1994, p. 10.

5. National Advisory Mental Health Council, p. 10.

6. Wyatt and Henter, p. 3.

7. Mrazek, Patricia J., and Robert J. Haggerty, *Reducing Risks for Mental Disorders: Frontiers for Preventive Intervention Research.* (Washington, D.C.: National Academy Press, 1994), pp. vi–vii.

8. National Institutes of Health, *A Plan for Prevention Research for the National Institute of Mental Health: A Report to the National Advisory Mental Health Council,* NIH publication no. 96-4093 (National Institutes of Health, 1996), p. 12.

9. Mrazek and Haggerty, p. 12.

10. National Advisory Mental Health Council, pp. 10–15.

11. Kandler, Kenneth S., and Scott R. Diehl, "The Genetics of Schizophrenia: A Current Genetic-Epidemiologic Perspective," in *Special Report: Schizophrenia 1993* (National Institute of Mental Health, 1993).

12. DeAngelis, Tori, "When Children Don't Bond with Parents," *APA Monitor,* June 1997.

13. "Psychologists Strive to Offset Effects of Maternal Depression on Young Children," *APA Monitor,* June 1997.

14. Beardslee, William, "Mental Disorders: Time to Consider Prevention" (Speech delivered at "Children & Families at Risk: Collaborating with Our Schools," the Tenth Annual Rosalynn Carter Symposium on Mental Health Policy, Atlanta, Ga., November 2–3, 1994).

15. National Advisory Mental Health Council, pp. 14–15.

16. Working in conjunction with the Florida Mental Health Institute of the University of South Florida and the Center for the Study of Social Policy.

17. The Carter Center, "The Case for Kids: Community Strategies for Children and Families: Promoting Positive Outcomes" (Symposium, Atlanta, Ga., February 14–16, 1996), pp. 23–24.

18. National Institutes of Health, p. 7.

19. Personal communication from Nelba Chavez, administrator of Substance Abuse and Mental Health Services Administration, April 17, 1995. Also, Substance Abuse and Mental Health Services Administration, "School-Based/School Linked Activities."

20. Carnegie Task Force on Meeting the Needs of Young Children, *Starting Points: Meeting the Needs of Our Youngest Children* (New York: Carnegie Corporation of New York, 1994), cited in Young, Mary Eming, *Early Child Development: Investing in the Future* (Washington, D.C.: The World Bank, 1996), p. 5.

21. Mrazek and Haggerty, p. 87.

22. Beardslee, p. 13.

23. Young, pp. 3–4.

24. Beardslee, p. 15.

25. Rosenberg, Mark, "Violence: Solutions Are at Hand" (Speech delivered at "Children & Families at Risk: Collaborating with Our Schools," the Tenth Annual Rosalynn Carter Symposium on Mental Health Policy, Atlanta, Ga., November 2–3, 1994), p. 23.

26. Elders, Joycelyn, "Protecting the Nation's Future" (Speech delivered at "Children & Families at Risk: Collaborating with Our Schools," the Tenth Annual Rosalynn Carter Symposium on Mental Health Policy, Atlanta, Ga., November 2–3, 1994), p. 31.

27. Kunin, Madeleine K., "Education Is the Gateway to the Future" (Speech delivered at "Children & Families at Risk: Collaborating with Our Schools," the Tenth Annual Rosalynn Carter Symposium on Mental Health Policy, Atlanta, Ga., November 2–3, 1994), p. 35.

28. Rodriguez, Gloria, "Programs that Work: A Multifaceted Approach" (Speech delivered at "Children & Families at Risk: Collaborating with Our Schools," the Tenth Annual Rosalynn Carter Symposium on Mental Health Policy, Atlanta, Ga., November 2–3, 1994), pp. 47–49.

29. Mrazek and Haggerty, p. 128.

30. Dr. John Gates is the former Georgia commissioner for Mental Health and Substance Abuse.

31. Gates, John, "Fostering Resiliency" (Speech delivered at "The Case for Kids: Community Strategies for Children and Families: Promoting Positive Outcomes," Carter Center symposium, Atlanta, Ga., February 14–16, 1996), p. 12. Based on the work of Benard, Bonnie, "Fostering Resiliency in Kids: Protective Factors in the Family, School, and Community," *Prevention Forum* 12 (1992): pp. 1–16.

32. Werner, Emily E., "Resilient Children," in E. M. Hetherington and R. D. Parke, eds., *Contemporary Readings in Child Psychology* (New York: McGraw-Hill, 1987).

33. Hamburg, David A., *Today's Children: Creating a Future for a Generation in Crisis* (New York: Random House, 1992).

34. Dr. Julius Richmond, pediatrician by profession, helped develop Head Start. He is the former Surgeon General of the U.S.

Chapter 11

1. Maurin, Judith T., and Carlene Barmann Boyd, "Burden of Mental Illness on the Family: A Critical Review," *Archives of Psychiatric Nursing* 4 (1990): p. 99.

2. Johnson, Dale L., "The Family's Experience of Living with Mental Illness," in Harriet P. Lefley and Dale L. Johnson, eds.,

Families as Allies in Treatment of the Mentally Ill: New Directions for Mental Health Professionals (Washington, D.C.: American Psychiatric Press, 1990), p. 35.

3. MacGregor, Peggy, "Grief: The Unrecognized Parental Response to Mental Illness in Children," *Social Work* 39 (1994): p. 164.
4. Titelman, D., and L. Psyk, "Grief, Guilt, and Identification in Siblings of Schizophrenic Individuals," *Bulletin of the Menninger Clinic* 55 (1991): p. 8.
5. MacGregor, p. 164.
6. Lindgren, Carolyn L., "The Caregiver Career," *Image: Journal of Nursing Scholarship* 25 (1993): p. 214.
7. Felder, Leonard, *When a Loved One Is Ill: How to Take Better Care of Your Loved One, Your Family, and Yourself* (New York: Plume/Penguin, 1991).
8. Nottingham, Jack A., David Haigler, David L. Smith, and Pam Davis, *Characteristics, Concerns, and Concrete Needs of Formal and Informal Caregivers: Understanding and Appreciating Their Marathon Existence* (Americus, Ga.: The Rosalynn Carter Institute for Human Development, 1993).
9. Horwitz, Allan V., and Susan C. Reinhard, "Ethnic Differences in Caregiving Duties and Burdens Among Parents and Siblings of Persons with Severe Mental Illnesses," *Journal of Health and Social Behavior* 36 (1995): pp. 138–50.
10. Woolis, Rebecca, *When Someone You Love Has a Mental Illness: A Handbook for Family, Friends, and Caregivers* (Los Angeles: J. P. Tarcher, 1991).
11. Styron, p. 76.
12. Stuart Perry is a member of the Georgia State Mental Health Consumer Network and a regional representative on the State Consumer Council for the Georgia Division of Mental Health, Mental Retardation, and Substance Abuse.
13. Celine Dion's "Because You Loved Me"; Stuart Perry substituted the word *caregivers* for *baby* in the original song.

Chapter 12

1. Paul Jay Fink's coauthor, Allan Tasman, is chair of the Department of Psychiatry and Behavioral Sciences at the University of Louisville School of Medicine. In *Stigma and Mental Illness,* Paul

Jay Fink and Allan Tasman, eds. (Washington, D.C.: American Psychiatric Press, 1992).

2. Goffman, Erving, *Stigma: Notes on the Management of Spoiled Identity* (Englewood Cliffs, N.J.: Prentice Hall, 1963).

3. Simon, Bennett, "Shame, Stigma, and Mental Illness in Ancient Greece," in *Stigma and Mental Illness,* Paul Jay Fink and Allan Tasman, eds. (Washington, D.C.: American Psychiatric Press, 1992).

4. Dain, Norman, "Madness and the Stigma of Sin in American Christianity," in *Stigma and Mental Illness.*

5. George Gerbner, Ph.D., dean emeritus and professor of communications, Annenberg School for Communications, University of Pennsylvania, in "Images that Hurt: Mental Illness in the Mass Media," *The Journal of the California Alliance of the Mentally Ill* 4, no. 1 (1993): p. 17.

6. William R. Dubin and Paul Jay Fink in *Stigma and Mental Illness.*

7. Medical director of Sheppard Pratt Hospital, Baltimore.

8. Gabbard, Glen O., and Krin Gabbard, "Cinematic Stereotypes Contributing to Stigmatization of Psychiatrists," in *Stigma and Mental Illness,* Paul Jay Fink and Allan Tasman, eds. (Washington, D.C.: American Psychiatric Press, 1992), pp. 113–26.

9. Dubin, William R., and Paul Jay Fink, "Effects of Stigma on Psychiatric Treatment," in *Stigma and Mental Illness,* p. 4.

10. Mental Health Association of Georgia *Messenger,* February 1997.

Epilogue

1. Quoted in Gold, p. 290.

2. Jamison, p. 196.

3. Goleman, Daniel, "Research on Brain Leads to Pursuit of Designer Drugs," *The New York Times,* November 19, 1996.

4. David Pickar is chief of the Experimental Therapeutics Branch, Division of Intramural Research Programs at NIMH.

5. Beardslee, p. 17.

6. Harvard Medical School, Department of Social Medicine, *World Mental Health: Problems and Priorities in Low-Income Countries* (New York: Oxford University Press, 1995).

References

Abraham, Dylan. "Getting Well Is Not a Race." *NAMI Advocate,* January/February 1997, p. 10.

Akbarian, Schahram, James J. Kim, Steven G. Potkin, et al. "Maldistribution of Interstitial Neurons in Prefrontal White Matter of the Brains of Schizophrenic Patients." *Archives of General Psychiatry* 53 (1996): pp. 425–35.

Albee, George W. "Revolutions and Counterrevolutions in Prevention." *American Psychologist* 51 (1996): pp. 1130–33.

Albee, George W., and Thomas P. Gullota, eds. *Issues in Children's and Families' Lives.* Vol. 6, *Primary Prevention Works.* Thousand Oaks, Calif.: Sage Publications, 1997.

Allen, Albert J., Henrietta L. Leonard, and Susan E. Swedo. "Case Study: A New Infection-Triggered Autoimmune Subtype of Pediatric OCD and Tourette's Syndrome." *Journal of the American Academy of Child and Adolescent Psychiatry* 34 (1995): pp. 307–11.

Alliance for the Mentally Ill of Pennsylvania. *How Pennsylvania Residents View Persons with Mental Illness.* Harrisburg, Pa.: Alliance for the Mentally Ill of Pennsylvania 1992.

American Psychiatric Association. *Decision Makers: Mental Illness Awareness Guide.* Washington, D.C.: American Psychiatric Association, Division of Public Affairs, 1995.

American Psychiatric Association. *Image Makers: Mental Illness Awareness Guide.* Washington, D.C.: American Psychiatric Association, Division of Public Affairs, 1993.

References

American Psychiatric Association. *Let's Talk Facts About Schizophrenia.* Washington, D.C.: American Psychiatric Association Division of Public Affairs, 1994.

American Public Health Association. *Helping Mentally Ill Homeless People: A Manual for Shelter Workers.* Washington, D.C.: American Public Health Association, 1989.

"Atlanta Communities Urged to See the Warning Signs of Mental Illness." *Mental Health Notes,* Mental Health Association of Metropolitan Atlanta, April 1992, p. 1.

Andreasen, Nancy C., Stephan Arndt, Victor Swayze II, et al. "Thalamic Abnormalities in Schizophrenia Visualized Through Magnetic Resonance Image Averaging." *Science* 266 (1994): pp. 294–99.

Andreasen, Nancy C., Laura Flashman, et al. "Regional Brain Abnormalities in Schizophrenia Measured with Magnetic Resonance Imaging." *Journal of the American Medical Association* 272 (1994): pp. 1763–69.

Andreasen, Nancy C., Daniel S. O'Leary, Ted Cizadlo, et al. "Schizophrenia and Cognitive Dysmetria: A Positron-Emission Tomography Study of Dysfunctional Prefrontal-Thalamic-Cerebellar Circuitry." *Proceedings of the National Academy of Science USA* 93 (1996): pp. 9985–90.

Anthony, William A. "Changing Visions, Changing Lives: New Revolutions." *The CAMI Statement* XIII, no. 1 (May/June 1993): p. 1.

Anxiety and Stress Disorders Institute of Maryland. *Panic Disorders: Guidelines for Loved Ones.* Baltimore, Md.: Anxiety and Stress Disorders Institute of Maryland, 1992.

Azar, Beth. "Environment Is Key to Serotonin Levels." *APA Monitor,* April 1997.

Azar, Beth. "Nature, Nurture: Not Mutually Exclusive." *APA Monitor,* May 1997.

Azar, Beth. "Research Reveals Clues to Who Suffers Panic Attacks." *APA Monitor,* December 1996, p. 23.

Bachrach, Leona L. "The Carter Commission's Contributions to Mental Health Service Planning." *Hospital and Community Psychiatry* 45 (1994): pp. 527–43.

Baron-Faust, Rita. *Mental Wellness for Women.* New York: William Morrow & Co., 1997.

Beardslee, William. "Mental Disorders: Time to Consider Prevention." Speech delivered at "Children & Families at Risk: Collaborating with

Our Schools." The Tenth Annual Rosalynn Carter Symposium on Mental Health Policy. Atlanta, Ga., November 2–3, 1994.

Beck, Aaron. *Love is Never Enough.* New York: Harper & Row, 1988.

Bellack, Alan S., and Kim T. Mueser. "Psychosocial Treatment for Schizophrenia." In *Special Report: Schizophrenia 1993.* National Institute of Mental Health, 1993.

Bello, Kenya Napper. "Acute Depression is a Disease . . . Not a Character Flaw." *Black Men Don't Commit Suicide,* Spring 1995, p. 1.

Bello, Kenya Napper. "Shakur's Unheard Cry." *Atlanta Journal-Constitution,* September 30, 1996.

Benard, Bonnie. "Fostering Resiliency in Kids: Protective Factors in the Family, School, and Community." *Prevention Forum* 12 (1992): pp. 1–16.

Blakeslee, Sandra. "Fear and Anger Heard Deep Inside the Brain." *The New York Times,* January 21, 1997.

Blakeslee, Sandra. "Studies Pinpoint Region of Brain Implicated in Tourette's Syndrome." *The New York Times,* September 17, 1996.

Bock, James. "A Personal Tragedy, A Nationwide Trend." *Baltimore Sun,* December 9, 1996.

Bourdon, Karen H., Donald S. Rae, et al. "National Prevalence and Treatment of Mental and Addictive Disorders." In *Mental Health, United States, 1994,* Center for Mental Health Services, R. W. Manderscheid and M. A. Sonnenschein, eds. DHHS publication no. (SMA)94-3000. Washington, D.C.: U.S. Government Printing Office, 1994.

Boutros-Ghali, Boutros. Speech delivered at the launch of "World Mental Health: Problems and Priorities in Low-Income Countries" symposium. New York, May 15, 1995.

Bower, B. "Working Memory May Fail in Schizophrenia." *Science News,* March 22, 1997.

Boyd, Robert S. "What's Going on Inside the Brain?" *The Orange County Register,* December 24, 1996.

Breakey, William R., Pamela J. Fischer, M. Kramer, et al. "Health and Mental Health Problems of Homeless Men and Women in Baltimore." *Journal of the American Medical Association* 262 (1989): pp. 1352–57.

Breakey, William R., Pamela J. Fischer, Gerald Nestadt, and Alan Romanoski. "Stigma and Stereotype: Homeless Mentally Ill Persons." In *Stigma and Mental Illness,* Paul Jay Fink and Allan Tasman, eds. Washington, D.C.: American Psychiatric Press, 1992.

References

Breier, Alan, et al. "Schizophrenia is Associated with Elevated Amphetamine-Induced Synaptic Dopamine Concentrations: Evidence from a Positron Emission Tomography Method." *Proceedings of the National Academy of Science* 94 (1997), pp. 2567–74.

Breiter, Hans C., Nancy Etcoff, et al. "Response and Habituation of the Human Amygdala During Visual Processing of Facial Expressions." *Neuron* 17 (1996): pp. 875–87.

Britton, Gene. "Hospital Sanitation Branded Deplorable by Mental Prober." *The Altanta Constitution,* August 6, 1959.

Brizendine, Louann. "The Devon Asylum: A Brief History of the Changing Concept of Mental Illness and Asylum Treatment." In *Stigma and Mental Illness,* Paul Jay Fink and Allan Tasman, eds. Washington, D.C.: American Psychiatric Press, 1992.

Buchanan, Robert W. "Clozapine: Efficacy and Safety." *Schizophrenia Bulletin* 21 (1995): pp. 579–91.

Burns, David D. *Feeling Good: The New Mood Therapy.* New York: Avon Books, 1992.

Caldwell, Bettye. "Early Intervention: A Crucial Component of Family Support." Speech delivered at "Children & Families at Risk: Collaborating with Our Schools." The Tenth Annual Rosalynn Carter Symposium on Mental Health Policy. Atlanta, Ga., November 2–3, 1994, pp. 24–26.

Canino, Ian A. "Latino Children and Adolescents: Who Are They?" *Idea & Information Exchange, 1995: Reaching Underserved Populations.* American Academy of Child and Adolescent Psychiatry and the American Psychiatric Association, Division of Public Affairs, Washington, D.C., 1995, p. 47.

Carnegie Task Force on Meeting the Needs of Young Children. *Starting Points: Meeting the Needs of Our Youngest Children.* New York: Carnegie Corporation of New York, 1994. Cited in Mary Eming Young, *Early Child Development: Investing in the Future.* Washington, D.C.: The World Bank, 1996.

The Carter Center. "The Case for Kids: Community Strategies for Children and Families: Promoting Positive Outcomes. Symposium at The Carter Center. Atlanta, Ga., February 14–16, 1996.

Carter, Jimmy, and Rosalynn Carter. *Everything to Gain: Making the Most of the Rest of Your Life.* New York: Random House, 1987.

Carter, Rosalynn. "Don't Slight Mental Health Benefits." *The Washington Post,* August 9, 1993.

References

Carter, Rosalynn. *First Lady from Plains.* New York: Fawcett/Ballantine, 1984.

Carter, Rosalynn. "A Positive Link of Mind and Body." *Los Angeles Times,* May 7, 1996.

Carter, Rosalynn. Statement before the Senate Subcommittee on Health and Science Research, Washington, D.C., February 7, 1979.

Carter, Rosalynn. "Women Leaders of the World Make Mental Health a Priority." *APA Monitor,* May 1997.

Carter, Rosalyn, with Susan K. Golant. *Helping Yourself Help Others.* New York: Times Books, 1996.

Centers for Disease Control and Prevention. "Attempted Suicide Among High-School Students—United States, 1990." *Morbidity and Mortality Weekly Report* 40 (September 20, 1991).

Centers for Disease Control and Prevention. "Youth Risk Behavior Surveillance—United States, 1995." CDC Surveillance Summaries. *Morbidity and Mortality Weekly Report* 45, no. SS-4 (September 27, 1996): p. 8.

Chen, Edwin, and Robert A. Rosenblatt. "Mental Health Provisions May Imperil Reform Bill." *Los Angeles Times,* April 23, 1996.

Congress of the United States, Office of Technology Assessment. *The Biology of Mental Disorders: New Developments in Neuroscience.* Document OTA-BA-538. Washington, D.C.: U.S. Government Printing Office, September 1992.

Coyle, Joseph T. "Glutamate and Schizophrenia's Symptoms." *Brain Work: The Neuroscience Newsletter* 7 (May/June 1997): pp. 4–5.

Cronkite, Kathy. *On the Edge of Darkness: Conversations About Conquering Depression.* New York: Delta Books, 1994.

Crossette, Barbara. "Noncommunicable Diseases Seen as a World Challenge." *The New York Times,* September 16, 1996.

Crow, T. J. "Prenatal Exposure to Influenza as a Cause of Schizophrenia: There Are Inconsistencies and Contradictions to the Evidence." *British Journal of Psychiatry* 164 (1994): pp. 588–92.

Culbertson, Frances M. "Depression and Gender: An International Review." *American Psychologist* 52 (1997): pp. 25–31.

Dain, Norman. "Madness and the Stigma of Sin in American Christianity." In *Stigma and Mental Illness,* Paul Jay Fink and Allan Tasman, eds. Washington, D.C.: American Psychiatric Press, 1992.

Damasio, Antonio R. "Towards a Neuropathology of Emotion and Mood." *Nature* 386 (1997): pp. 769–70.

References

The Dana Alliance for Brain Initiatives. *Brain Research for the Life of Your Mind: Progress and Promise.* Washington, D.C.: The Dana Alliance for Brain Initiatives, 1996.

The Dana Alliance for Brain Initiatives. *Grey Matters: A Conversation with Art Buchwald, William Styron, and Mike Wallace.* Audiotape. Washington, D.C.: The Dana Alliance for Brain Initiatives, 1996.

DeAngelis, Tori. "Chromosomes Contain Clues to Schizophrenia." *APA Monitor,* January 1997, p. 26.

DeAngelis, Tori. "When Children Don't Bond with Parents." *APA Monitor,* June 1997.

Drevets, Wayne C., and Kelly Botteron. "Neuroimaging in Psychiatry." In *Adult Psychiatry,* Samuel B. Guze. ed. New York: Moseby, 1997.

Drevets, Wayne C., Joseph L. Price, Joseph R. Simpson, et al. "Subgenual Prefrontal Cortex Abnormalities in Mood Disorders." *Nature* 386 (1997): pp. 824–27.

Drevets, Wayne C., Tom O. Videen, Joseph L. Price, et al. "A Functional Anatomical Study of Unipolar Depression." *Journal of Neuroscience* 12 (1992): pp. 3628–41.

Dubin, William R., and Paul Jay Fink. "Effects of Stigma on Psychiatric Treatment." In *Stigma and Mental Illness,* Paul Jay Fink and Allan Tasman, eds. Washington, D.C.: American Psychiatric Press, 1992.

Eakes, Georgene G. "Chronic Sorrow: The Lived Experience of Parents of Chronically Mentally Ill Individuals." *Archives of Psychiatric Nursing* 9 (1995): pp. 77–84.

Elders, Joycelyn. "Protecting the Nation's Future." Speech delivered at "Children & Families at Risk: Collaborating with Our Schools." The Tenth Annual Rosalynn Carter Symposium on Mental Health Policy. Atlanta, Ga., November 2–3, 1994, pp. 29–31.

Employee Benefit and Research Institute. *Analysis of the March 1995 Consumer Population Survey: Sources of Health Insurance and Characteristics of the Uninsured.* Baltimore, Md.: Employee Benefit and Research Institute Publications, 1996.

"Family Therapy May Aid Recovery from Manic Depression." *The New York Times,* May 20, 1997.

Farina, Amerigo, Jeffrey D. Fisher, and Edward H. Fisher. "Societal Factors in the Problems Faced by Deinstitutionalized Psychiatric Patients." In *Stigma and Mental Illness,* Paul Jay Fink and Allan Tasman, eds. Washington, D.C.: American Psychiatric Press, 1992.

References

Felder, Leonard. *When a Loved One Is Ill: How to Take Better Care of Your Loved One, Your Family, and Yourself.* New York: Plume/Penguin, 1991.

Fink, Paul Jay, and Allan Tasman, eds. *Stigma and Mental Illness.* Washington, D.C.: American Psychiatric Press, 1992.

First, Michael B., Allen Frances, and Harold Alan Pincus. *DSM-IV™ Handbook of Differential Diagnosis.* Washington, D.C.: American Psychiatric Press, 1995.

Fish, Barbara. "Neurobiological Antecedents of Schizophrenia in Childhood." *Archives of General Psychiatry* 34 (1977): pp. 1297–313.

Fox, Candace Smith. "The Most Powerful Family Intervention—The Letter." *Contra Costa AMI Newsletter,* November/December 1996.

Frazier, Jean A., et al. "Brain Anotomic Magnetic Resonance Imaging in Childhood Onset Schizophrenia," *Archives of General Psychiatry* 53 (1996): pp. 617–24.

Freud, Anna. *War and Children.* Greenwood Publishing Group, 1993.

Freudenberger, Herbert J. "Recognizing and Dealing with Burnout." In *The Professional and Family Caregiver—Dilemmas, Rewards and New Directions,* Jack A. Nottingham and Joanne Nottingham, eds. Americus, Ga.: The Rosalynn Carter Institute for Human Development, 1990.

Frith, Chris. "Functional Imaging and Cognitive Abnormalities." *The Lancet* 346 (1995): pp. 615–20.

Gabbard, Glen O., and Krin Gabbard. "Cinematic Stereotypes Contributing to Stigmatization of Psychiatrists." In *Stigma and Mental Illness,* Paul Jay Fink and Allan Tasman, eds. Washington, D.C.: American Psychiatric Press, 1992.

Gates, John. "Fostering Resiliency." Speech delivered at "The Case for Kids: Community Strategies for Children and Families: Promoting Positive Outcomes." Symposium at The Carter Center. Atlanta, Ga., February 14–16, 1996, pp. 12–14.

Gates, John, and Judy Fitzgerald. "Carter Center Focuses on Reducing Problems Confronting Children and Families at Risk." *NMHA Prevention Update* 6 (Spring/Summer 1995): p. 1.

Gerbner, George. "Images that Hurt: Mental Illness in the Mass Media." *Journal of the California Alliance for the Mentally Ill* 4, no. 1 (1993): p. 17.

Gilbert, Susan. "Lag Seen in Aid for Depression." *The New York Times,* January 22, 1997.

Ginns, Edward, J. Ott, and Janice Egeland, et al. "A Genome-Wide Search for Chromosomal Loci Linked to Bipolar Affective Disorder in the Old Amish Order." *Nature Genetics* 12 (1996): pp. 431–35.

Goetinck, Sue. "The Biology Behind Suicide: Brain Chemistry Examined to Help Find People at Risk." *Dallas Morning News,* December 23, 1996, p. 6D.

Goffman, Erving. *Stigma: Notes on the Management of Spoiled Identity.* Englewood Cliffs, N.J.: Prentice Hall, 1963.

Golant, Mitch, and Susan K. Golant. *What to Do When Someone You Love Is Depressed.* New York: Villard Books, 1996.

Gold, Mark S., and Lois B. Morris. *The Good News About Depression.* New York: Bantam Books, 1995.

Goleman, Daniel. "Brain Images Show the Neural Basis of Addiction as It Is Happening." *The New York Times,* August 13, 1996.

Goleman, Daniel. "Evidence Mounting for Role of Fetal Damage in Schizophrenia." *The New York Times,* May 28, 1996.

Goleman, Daniel. "Making Room on the Couch for Culture." *The New York Times,* December 5, 1995.

Goleman, Daniel. "Research on Brain Leads to Pursuit of Designer Drugs." *The New York Times,* November 19, 1996.

Goodman, W. K., C. J. McDougle, et al. "Beyond the Serotonin Hypothesis: A Role for Dopamine in Some Forms of Obsessive-Compulsive Disorder." *Journal of Clinical Psychiatry* 51 (1990): pp. 36–43.

Govig, Stewart. "Wilderness Journal: Parental Engagement with Young Adult Mental Illness." *Word & World* 9 (1989): pp. 147–53.

Grady, Denise. "Brain-Tied Gene Defect May Explain Why Schizophrenics Hear Voices." *The New York Times,* January 21, 1997.

Greist, John H., and James W. Jefferson. *Depression and Its Treatment,* rev. ed. Washington, D.C.: American Psychiatric Press, 1992.

Hamburg, David A. *Today's Children: Creating a Future for a Generation in Crisis.* New York: Random House, 1992.

Harvard Medical School, Department of Social Medicine. *World Mental Health: Problems and Priorities in Low-Income Countries.* New York: Oxford University Press, 1995.

Hollister, J. Megginson, Peter Laing, and Sarnoff A. Mednick. "Rhesus Incompatibility as a Risk Factor for Schizophrenia in Male Adults." *Archives of General Psychiatry* 53 (1996): pp. 19–24.

Horwitz, Allan V., and Susan C. Reinhard. "Ethnic Differences in Caregiving Duties and Burdens Among Parents and Siblings of Persons with Severe Mental Illnesses." *Journal of Health and Social Behavior* 36 (1995): pp. 138–50.

Hymowitz, Carol, and Ellen Joan Pollock. "Psychobattle: Cost-Cutting Firms Monitor Couch Time as Therapists Fret." *The Wall Street Journal,* July 13, 1995, p. 1.

Jamison, Kay Redfield. *An Unquiet Mind: A Memoir of Moods and Madness.* New York: Knopf, 1995.

Johnson, Dale L. "The Family's Experience of Living with Mental Illness." In *Families as Allies in Treatment of the Mentally Ill: New Directions for Mental Health Professionals,* Harriet P. Lefley and Dale L. Johnson, eds. Washington, D.C.: American Psychiatric Press, 1990.

Johnstone, E. C., et al. "The Harrow (1975–1985) Study of the Disabilities and Circumstances of Schizophrenic Patients." *British Journal of Psychiatry* 159, suppl. 13 (1991): pp. 34–36, 44–46.

Kandler, Kenneth S., and Scott R. Diehl. "The Genetics of Schizophrenia: A Current Genetic-Epidemiologic Perspective." In *Special Report: Schizophrenia 1993.* National Institute of Mental Health, 1993.

Kanowski, S. "Depression in the Elderly: Clinical Considerations and Therapeutic Approaches." *Journal of Clinical Psychiatry* 55 (1994): pp. 166–73.

Karno, Marvin. "The Prevalence of Mental Disorder Among Persons of Mexican American Birth or Origin." In *Latino Mental Health: Current Research and Policy Perspectives,* Cynthia Telles and Marvin Karno, eds. Los Angeles: Neuropsychiatric Institute, University of California, Los Angeles (1994): p. 3.

Karno, Marvin, and A. Morales. "Community Mental Health Service for Mexican-Americans in a Metropolis." *Comprehensive Psychiatry* 12 (1971): pp. 116–21.

Kass, Fredric. "Mental Illness and Homelessness." *Psychiatric News,* October 6, 1989: p. 3.

Katz, Ira R. "Prevention of Suicide Through Education on Late Life Depression." Testimony before the Senate Select Committee on Aging, Washington, D.C., July 30, 1996.

Kelleher, Kathleen. "Do-It-Yourself Love Potion Explains a Lot." *Los Angeles Times,* June 12, 1997, p. E3.

References

Kelleher, Kelly. "Mental Health in Primary Care: Major Trends and Issues." *Policy in Perspective.* The Mental Health Policy Resource Center, June 1995, p. 1.

Kelleher, Susan. "Attending to A.D.D." *The Orange County Register,* December 25, 1996.

Kessler, Ronald C., Katherine A. McGonagle, et al. "Lifetime and 12-month Prevalence of DSM-IIIR Psychiatric Disorders in the United States: Results from the National Comorbidity Study." *Archives of General Psychiatry* 51 (1994): pp. 8–19.

Kilts, Clinton D., Department of Psychiatry, Emory University, Atlanta, Ga. Personal communication, 1996.

Klein, Rachel Gittleman. "Is Panic Disorder Associated with Childhood Separation Anxiety Disorder?" *Clinical Neuropharmacology* 18, suppl. 2 (1995): pp. S7–S14.

Knitzer, Jane. *Unclaimed Children: The Failure of Public Responsibility to Children and Adolescents in Need of Mental Health Services.* Washington, D.C.: Children's Defense Fund, 1982.

Kolata, Gina. "Which Comes First: Depression or Heart Disease?" *The New York Times,* January 14, 1997.

Koyanagi, Chris, and Howard H. Goldman. "The Quiet Success of the National Plan for the Chronically Mentally Ill." *Hospital and Community Psychiatry* 42 (1991): pp. 1–7.

Kramer, Peter D. *Listening to Prozac.* New York: Viking, 1993.

Kunde, Diana. "Employers Offer Help to Depressed Workers." *Sunday Oregonian,* March 12, 1995, p. B1.

Kunin, Madeleine K. "Education Is the Gateway to the Future." Speech delivered at "Children & Families at Risk: Collaborating with Our Schools." The Tenth Annual Rosalynn Carter Symposium on Mental Health Policy. Atlanta, Ga., November 2–3, 1994, p. 34–35.

Lamy, R. E. "Social Consequence of Mental Illness." *Journal of Consulting Clinical Psychology* 30 (1966): pp. 450–55.

Landers, Ann. "Mental Illness Is Often a Treatable Condition." *Los Angeles Times,* September 4, 1997, p. E3.

Lavin, Don, and Andrea Everett. *Working on the Dream: A Guide to Career Planning and Job Success.* Spring Lake Park, Minn.: Rise, Inc., 1996.

Leary, Warren E. "Depression Travels in Disguise with Other Illnesses." *The New York Times,* January 17, 1996.

Lebowitz, Barry D. " 'Depression is Diabetes'—Demanding Parity for Mental Health." *Aging Today,* July/August 1994.

Lebowitz, Barry D. *Fact Sheet: How Physical and Mental Health Interact in Older Persons.* NIMH Mental Disorders of Aging Research Branch; Alcohol, Drug Abuse and Mental Health Administration; Public Health Service; U.S. Department of Health and Human Services, July 1991.

Lefley, Harriet P. "Awakenings and Recovery: Learning the Beat of a Different Drummer." *The Journal of the California Alliance for the Mentally Ill* 7 (July 1996): pp. 4–6.

Lefley, Harriet P. "The Stigmatized Family." In *Stigma and Mental Illness,* Paul Jay Fink and Allan Tasman, eds. Washington, D.C.: American Psychiatric Press, 1992.

Leonard, Henrietta L., Marge C. Lenane, and Susan E. Swedo. "Obsessive Compulsive Disorder." *Child and Adolescent Psychiatric Clinics of North America* 2 (1993): pp. 655–66.

Leonard, Henrietta L., Susan E. Swedo, Judith L. Rapoport, et al. "Treatment of Obsessive-Compulsive Disorder with Clomipramine and Desipramine in Children and Adolescents." *Archives of General Psychiatry* 46 (1989): pp. 1088–92.

Leshner, Alan. *Outcasts on Main Street: A Report of the Federal Task Force on Homelessness and Severe Mental Illness.* Rockville, Md.: National Institute of Mental Health, Office of Programs for the Mentally Ill, 1992.

Lewin, Tamar. "Questions of Privacy Roil Arena of Psychotherapy." *The New York Times,* May 22, 1996.

Lindgren, Carolyn L. "The Caregiver Career." *Image: Journal of Nursing Scholarship* 25 (1993): p. 214.

Link, Bruce G., Francis T. Cullen, Jerold Mirotznik, and Elmer Streuning. "The Consequences of Stigma for Persons with Mental Illness: Evidence from the Social Sciences." In *Stigma and Mental Illness,* Paul Jay Fink and Allan Tasman, eds. Washington, D.C.: American Psychiatric Press, 1992.

MacGregor, Peggy. "Grief: The Unrecognized Parental Response to Mental Illness in Children." *Social Work* 39 (1994): pp. 160–66.

"Majority of Homeless People Found to be Mentally Ill." *Psychiatric News,* October 6, 1989, p. 11.

Manderscheid, Ron, and Mary Anne Sonnenschein. *Mental Health, United States, 1996.* Center for Mental Health Services of the Substance Abuse and Mental Health Services Administration, U.S. Department of Health and Human Services, 1997.

"Marker Identified for Children at Risk for OCD After Strep." *Psychiatric News,* January 17, 1997.

References

Maurin, Judith T., and Carlene Barmann Boyd. "Burden of Mental Illness on the Family: A Critical Review." *Archives of Psychiatric Nursing* 4 (1990): pp. 99–107.

Marquis, Julie. "Erasing the Line Between Mental and Physical Ills." *Los Angeles Times,* October 15, 1996, p. 1A.

McGrath, E., G. P. Keita, Bonnie Strickland, et al. *Women and Depression: Risk Factors and Treatment Issues.* Washington, D.C.: American Psychological Association, 1990.

McGuffin, Peter, Michael J. Owen, and Anne E. Farmer. "Genetic Basis of Schizophrenia." *The Lancet* 346 (1995): pp. 678–82.

Mednick, S. A., R. A. Machon, M. O. Huttunen, et al. "Adult Schizophrenia Following Prenatal Exposure to an Influenza Epidemic." *Archives of General Psychiatry* 45 (1988): pp. 189–92.

Mental Health Policy Resource Center. "Themes and Variations: Mental Health and Substance Abuse Policy in the Making." *Policy in Perspective,* April 1996.

Miller, Andy. "Columbus Firms Champion Mental Health Coverage." *Mental Health Association of Georgia Messenger,* May 1997, p. 1.

Moldawsky, Stanley. "Managed Care and Psychotherapy are Incompatible." *APA Monitor,* July 1997, p. 24.

Moller, Mary D. "Learning from the Awakening." *The Journal of the California Alliance of the Mentally Ill* 7 (July 1996): pp. 10–11.

Mrazek, Patricia J., and Robert J. Haggerty, eds. *Reducing Risks for Mental Disorders: Frontiers for Preventive Intervention Research.* Washington, D.C.: National Academy Press, 1994.

Murray, Christopher J. L., and Alan D. Lopez, eds. *Summary: The Global Burden of Disease.* Cambridge, Mass.: Harvard University Press, 1996.

National Advisory Mental Health Council. *Basic Behavioral Science Research for Mental Health: A National Investment.* NIH publication no. 95-3682. U.S. Department of Health and Human Services, National Institute of Mental Health, 1995.

National Advisory Mental Health Council. *National Plan for Research on Child and Adolescent Mental Disorders.* DHHS publication no. (ADM) 90-1683. U.S. Department of Health and Human Services, Alcohol, Drug Abuse, and Mental Health Administration, 1990.

National Alliance for the Mentally Ill. *Family Perspectives on Meeting the Needs for Care of Severely Mentally Ill Relatives: A National Survey,* funded by the John D. and Catherine T. MacArthur Foundation. Arlington, Va.: National Alliance for the Mentally Ill, 1991.

National Coalition for the Homeless. "Why Are People Homeless?" *NCH Fact Sheet #1.* Washington, D.C.: National Coalition for the Homeless, 1996.

National Coalition of Hispanic Health and Human Service Organizations. *Growing Up Hispanic.* Vol. II, *National Chartbook.* Washington, D.C.: National Coalition of Hispanic Health and Human Service Organizations, 1995.

National Coalition of Hispanic Health and Human Service Organizations. *Mental Health of the Immigrant Child: A Report to the Annie E. Casey Foundation.* Washington, D.C.: National Coalition of Hispanic Health and Human Service Organizations, 1995.

National Institutes of Health. *A Plan for Prevention Research for the National Institute of Mental Health: A Report to the National Advisory Mental Health Council.* National Institute of Health, NIH publication no. 96-4093, 1996.

National Institute of Mental Health. Memorandum from Alan Leshner, deputy director, concerning cost-effectiveness of mental health services, March 1993.

National Institute of Mental Health. *The Neuroscience of Mental Health II.* NIH publication no. 95-4000. Rockville, Md.: U.S. National Institutes of Health, National Institute of Mental Health, 1995.

National Institute of Mental Health. *Schizophrenia: Questions and Answers.* DHHS publication no. (ADM) 86-1457. U.S. Department of Health and Human Services, National Institute of Mental Health, reprinted, 1990.

National Institute of Mental Health, Depression Awareness, Recognition, and Treatment (D/ART) Program. *Sex Differences in Depressive Disorders: A Review of Recent Research.* U.S. Department of Health and Human Services, National Institute of Mental Health, 1987.

Nelson, Jack. "Disturbed Georgia Children Get Clinic, Private Help." *The Atlanta Constitution,* July 19, 1959.

Nelson, Jack. "Do Patients Just Mark Time in Milledgeville Slack?" *The Atlanta Constitution,* March 15, 1959.

Nelson, Jack. "House Mental Unit Asks 5-Year Plan." *The Atlanta Constitution,* June 19, 1959.

Nelson, Jack. "Ineligibles Given Surgery; Mental Patients Wait Turns." *The Atlanta Constitution,* March 26, 1959.

Nelson, Jack. "Mental Hub Slated Here." *The Atlanta Journal,* August 27, 1960.

Nelson, Jack. "Milledgeville Probe Hears Key Figures." *The Atlanta Constitution,* March 16, 1959.

Nelson, Jack. "Psychiatrists' Extra Duty Frees 25 at Milledgeville." *The Atlanta Journal,* March 20, 1961.

Nelson, Jack. "State Mental Care for Youth Lagging." *The Atlanta Journal,* August 7, 1960.

Nelson, Jack. "Unapproved Drugs Given Mental Cases." *The Atlanta Constitution,* March 5, 1959.

Nelson, Jack. "Use of Drugs, Anesthesia Investigated." *The Atlanta Constitution,* March 18, 1959.

Nolen-Hoeksema, Susan K. *Sex Differences in Depression.* Stanford, Calif.: Stanford University Press, 1990.

Nottingham, Jack A., David Haigler, David L. Smith, and Pam Davis. *Characteristics, Concerns, and Concrete Needs of Formal and Informal Caregivers: Understanding and Appreciating Their Marathon Existence.* Americus, Ga.: The Rosalynn Carter Institute for Human Development, 1993.

Palmer, Jodi White. "Woman Wins Battle with Mental Illness." *The Macon Telegraph,* October 5, 1996.

Pear, Robert. "Employers Told to Accommodate the Mentally Ill." *The New York Times,* April 30, 1997.

Pearson, Jane L. Testimony before the Senate Select Committee on Aging, Washington, D.C., July 30, 1996.

Pennisi, Elizabeth. "Key Protein Found for Brain's Dopamine-Producing Neurons." *Science Magazine Online,* April 11, 1997.

Perlmutter, Richard A. "A Clinical Family Approach to Anxiety Disorders." *ADAA Reporter,* Spring 1997, p. 2.

Pines, Marion. "Programs That Work: Taking Services to Families." Speech delivered at "Children & Families at Risk: Collaborating with Our Schools." The Tenth Annual Rosalynn Carter Symposium on Mental Health Policy. Atlanta, Ga., November 2–3, 1994, pp. 40–43.

PJB Publications. *Pharmacoprojects.* Surrey, England: PJB Publications, 1992.

Potter, Pat, and Gordon Roberts. "Mind Without Hope Thinks of Fire." *The Atlanta Constitution,* August 24, 1960.

Potter, Pat, and Gordon Roberts. "State Youth Mental Care Is Lagging." *The Atlanta Constitution,* August 22, 1960.

President's Commission on Mental Health. *The Report to the President from the President's Commission on Mental Health, 1978.* Document 040-

000–00390-8. Washington, D.C.: U.S. Government Printing Office, 1978.

"Psychologists Strive to Offset Effects of Maternal Depression on Young Children." *APA Monitor,* June 1997.

Radcliffe, Donnie. "A Former First Lady's Second Opinion." *The Washington Post,* June 24, 1993.

Raleigh, Fred. "A New Beginning." *The Journal of the California Alliance of the Mentally Ill* 7 (July 1996): pp. 7–9.

Rautktis, Mary Elizabeth, Gary F. Koeske, and Olga Tereshko. "Negative Social Interactions, Distress, and Depression Among Those Caring for a Seriously and Persistently Mentally Ill Relative." *American Journal of Community Psychology* 23 (1995): pp. 279–99.

Real, Terrence. *I Don't Want to Talk About It.* New York: Scribners, 1997.

Recer, Paul. "Gene Triggers, Wanes Anxiety." *Los Angeles Times AP Online, Health,* December 1, 1996.

Regier, Darrel A., Mary E. Farmer, Donald S. Rae, et al. "Comorbidity of Mental Disorders with Alcohol and Other Drug Abuse: Results from the Epidemiologic Catchment Area (ECA) Study." *Journal of the American Medical Association* 264 (1990): pp. 2511–18.

Reifman, A., and R. J. Wyatt. "Lithium: A Brake in the Rising Cost of Mental Illness." *Archives of General Psychiatry* 37 (1980): pp. 385–88.

Reiss, David. "The Prevention of Mental Disorders: A National Research Agenda." National Institute of Mental Health, 1994. Quoted in "MH Coalition Highlights Value of Prevention, Research, Training." *Psychiatric News,* January 7, 1994, p. 10.

"Research Begins to Yield Understanding of Childhood Schizophrenia." *Psychiatric News,* January 17, 1997.

Reveley, A. M., M. A. Reveley, et al. "Cerebral Ventricular Size in Twins Discordant for Schizophrenia." *The Lancet* ii (1982): pp. 540–41.

Rex, John. "Oh My Son: A Sermon." Delivered at the Unitarian Universalist Fellowship of Fredricksburg, Va., September 15, 1995.

Rice, D. P., S. Kelman, et al. *The Economic Costs of Alcohol and Drug Abuse and Mental Illness: 1985.* DHHS publication no. (ADM) 90-1694. Department of Health and Human Services, Center for Mental Health Services, 1990.

Rice, D. P., and L. K. Miller. *The Economic Burden of Mental Disorders.* Rockville, Md.: Substance Abuse and Mental Health Services Administration, 1993.

Riger, Stephanie, and Pat Gilligan. "Women in Management: An Exploration of Competency Paradigms." *American Psychologist* 35 (1980): pp. 902–11.

Risby, Emile, Deane Donnigan, and Charles Nemeroff. "Formulary Considerations for Treating Psychiatric Disorders: Schizophrenia." *Formulary* 32 (1997): pp. 142–55.

Risby, Emile, Deane Donnigan, and Charles Nemeroff. "Psychotherapeutic Considerations for Psychiatric Disorders: Depression." *Formulary* 32 (1997): pp. 46–59.

Ritter, Malcolm. "Study Finds No Sign 'Anxiety Gene.' " *Los Angeles Times AP Online, Health,* May 1, 1997.

Robins, Lee N., Ben Z. Locke, and Darrel A. Regier. "An Overview of Psychiatric Disorders in America." In *Psychiatric Disorders in America: The Epidemiologic Catchment Area Study,* Lee N. Robins and Darrel A. Regier, eds. New York: Free Press, 1991.

Rodriguez, Gloria. "Programs That Work: A Multifaceted Approach." Speech delivered at "Children & Families at Risk: Collaborating with Our Schools." The Tenth Annual Rosalynn Carter Symposium on Mental Health Policy. Atlanta, Ga., November 2–3, 1994, pp. 47–49.

Rosen, Laura Epstein, and Xavier F. Amador. *When Someone You Love Is Depressed.* New York: Free Press, 1996.

Rosenberg, Mark. "Violence: Solutions Are at Hand." Speech delivered at "Children & Families at Risk: Collaborating with Our Schools." The Tenth Annual Rosalynn Carter Symposium on Mental Health Policy. Atlanta, Ga., November 2–3, 1994, pp. 21–23.

Rosenthal, A. M. "Park Avenue Lady." *The New York Times,* November 23, 1996.

Rosenthal, N. E., D. A. Sack, J. C. Gillin, et al. "Seasonal Affective Disorder: Description of the Syndrome and Preliminary Findings with Light Therapy." *Archives of General Psychiatry* 41 (1984): pp. 72–78.

Ross, Jerilyn. *Triumph over Fear: A Book of Help and Hope for People with Anxiety, Panic Attacks, and Phobias.* New York: Bantam Books, 1994.

Rue, David. "Depression and Suicidal Behavior Among Asian Whiz Kids." In *The Emerging Generation of Korean-Americans,* Ho-Youn and Shin Kim, eds. Seoul, Korea: Lyung Hee University Press, 1993.

Rue, David. "Understanding Shame in Asian American Youths." In *Idea & Information Exchange, 1995: Reaching Underserved Populations,* American Academy of Child and Adolescent Psychiatry.

References

Rutter, M. "Resilience in the Face of Adversity: Protective Factors and Resistance to Psychiatric Disorder." *British Journal of Psychiatry* 147 (1985): pp. 598–611.

SAMHSA. *Mental Illness Is Not a Full-Time Job.* DHHS publication no. (SMA) 96-3102. U.S. Department of Health and Human Services, Substance Abuse and Mental Health Services Administration, 1996.

Sartorius, N. "WHO's Work on the Epidemiology of Mental Disorders." *Social Psychiatry* 1 (1993): pp. 30–31.

Schooler, Carmi, et al. "A Time Course Analysis of Stroop Interference and Facilitation: Comparing Normal Individuals and Individuals with Schizophrenia." *Journal of Experimental Psychology: General* 126 (March 1997).

Schwartz, Jeffrey M. *Brain Lock: Free Yourself from Obsessive-Compulsive Behavior.* New York: HarperCollins, 1996.

Sedvall, Goren, and Lars Farde. "Chemical Brain Anatomy in Schizophrenia." *The Lancet* 346 (1995): pp. 743–49.

Sharma, Tonmoy. "Schizophrenia: Recent Advances in Psychopharmacology." *British Journal of Hospital Medicine* 55 (1996): pp. 194–98.

Silbersweig, David, and E. Stern. "Functional Neuroimaging of Hallucinations in Schizophrenia: Toward an Integration of Bottom-Up and Top-Down Approaches." *Molecular Psychiatry* 1 (1996): pp. 367–75.

Silbersweig, David, E. Stern, C. Frith, et al. "A Functional Neuroanatomy of Hallucinations in Schizophrenia." *Nature* 378 (1995): pp. 176–79.

Simmons, Adelle. "All Children Are Our Children." Speech delivered at "Children & Families at Risk: Collaborating with Our Schools." The Tenth Annual Rosalynn Carter Symposium on Mental Health Policy. Atlanta, Ga., November 2–3, 1994, pp. 9–12.

Simon, Bennett. "Shame, Stigma, and Mental Illness in Ancient Greece." In *Stigma and Mental Illness,* Paul Jay Fink and Allan Tasman, eds. Washington, D.C.: American Psychiatric Press, 1992.

Sleek, Scott. "When Depression Lurks Beneath an Addiction." *American Psychological Association Monitor,* January 1997, p. 33.

Sperling, Dan. "Families Struggle with Kids' Hyperactive Behavior." *USA Today,* February 6, 1990, p. 4D.

Spurlock, Jeanne. "African American Families." In *Idea & Information Exchange, 1995: Reaching Underserved Populations,* American Academy of Child and Adolescent Psychiatry, Washington, D.C., p. 55.

References

Steinberg, Neil. "Drug Firms Want to Market Antidepressants for Kids." *Sun-Times* (Chicago), April 7, 1997.

Strauss, John S. "Pulling Themselves Together." *The Journal of the California Alliance of the Mentally Ill* 7 (July 1996): pp. 19–20.

Stroul, Beth A. *Children's Mental Health: Creating Systems of Care in a Changing Society.* Baltimore, Md.: Paul H. Brookes Publishing, 1996.

Styron, William. *Darkness Visible: A Memoir of Madness.* New York: Vintage Books, 1992.

Substance Abuse and Mental Health Services Administration. "School-Based/School Linked Activities."

Suddath, R. L., G. W. Christison, et al. "Cerebral Anatomical Abnormalities in Monozygotic Twins Discordant for Schizophrenia." *New England Journal of Medicine* 322 (1990): pp. 789–94.

Susser, E., and R. Neugebauer, et al. "Schizophrenia after Prenatal Exposure to Famine." *Archives of General Psychiatry* 53 (1996): pp. 25–31.

Swedo, Susan E. "Bad News and Good News About Obsessive-Compulsive Disorder." *Contemporary Pediatrics,* September 1989, pp. 130–51.

Swedo, Susan E. "Sydenham's Chorea: A Model for Childhood Autoimmune Neuropsychiatric Disorders." *Journal of the American Medical Association* 272 (1994): pp. 1788–91.

Swedo, Susan E., and Henrietta Leonard. *It's Not All in Your Head: The Real Causes and the Newest Solutions to Women's Most Common Health Problems.* San Francisco: HarperSanFrancisco, 1996.

Talan, Jamie. "Depression Forecasts: Researchers Focus on Brain Scans and Drug Therapy." *Newsday,* March 11, 1997.

Talan, Jamie. "Schizophrenia 'Trigger' Described/Brain Chemical Tests Clue to Psychosis." *Newsday,* March 19, 1997.

Talan, Jamie. "Where Fear Resides: Scientists are Mapping the Area of the Brain That Regulates This Response." *Newsday,* March 11, 1997.

Tanoye, Elyse. "Antidepressant Makers Study Kids' Market." *The Wall Street Journal,* April 4, 1997.

Terkelson, K. G. "The Meaning of Mental Illness to the Family." In *Families of the Mentally Ill,* A. B. Hatfield and H. P. Lefley, eds. New York: Guilford Press, 1987.

Titelman, D., and L. Psyk. "Grief, Guilt, and Identification in Siblings of Schizophrenic Individuals." *Bulletin of the Menninger Clinic* 55 (1991): pp. 72–84.

References

Torrey, E. F. *Hidden Victims: An Eight Stage Healing Process for Families and Friends of the Mentally Ill*. New York: Doubleday, 1988.

Torrey, E. F. *Out of the Shadows*. New York: John Wiley & Sons, Inc., 1997.

U.S. Department of Health and Human Services. *Justification of Estimates for Appropriations Committees, Fiscal Year 1997*. Public Health Service, National Institutes of Health–Volume IV; National Institute of Mental Health, 1997.

U.S. Department of Health and Human Services. *National Plan for Research on Child and Adolescent Mental Disorders*. ADM publication no. (ADM) 90-1683. Washington, D.C.: Public Health Service; Alcohol, Drug Abuse, and Mental Health Administration, 1990.

U.S. Department of Health and Human Services Steering Committee on the Chronically Mentally Ill. *Toward a National Plan for the Chronically Mentally Ill*. Washington, D.C.: Public Health Service, 1980.

Umland, Beth, and Foster Higgins. "Foster Higgins National Survey: Trends and Behavioral Benefits." *Behavioral Healthcare Tomorrow*, June 1997, p. 58.

Valleni-Basile, Laura A., Carol Z. Garrison, Kirby L. Jackson, et al. "Frequency of Obsessive-Compulsive Disorder in a Community Sample of Young Adolescents." *Journal of the American Academy of Child and Adolescent Psychiatry* 33 (1994): p. 782.

Varner, Bill. "Depression, Suicide Prey on the Elderly." *USA Today*, October 8, 1996, p. 2A.

Vitiello, Benedetto, and Peter S. Jensen. "Psychopharmacology in Children and Adolescents: Current Problems, Future Prospects: Summary Notes on the 1995 NIMH-FDA Conference." *Journal of Child and Adolescent Psychopharmacology* 5 (1995): pp. 5–7.

Vobejda, Barbara, and Judith Havemann. "Large U.S. Cities Target Homeless, Advocates Say." *The Washington Post*, December 12, 1996, p. A23.

Volz, Joe. "Depression Treatable Quickly and Effectively." *Plain Dealer* (Cleveland), February 21, 1995, p. 10E.

Wahl, Otto F. "Messages About Mental Illness from the Serial Killer Movie." *Journal of the California Alliance for the Mentally Ill* 4 (1993): p. 41.

Walker, Elaine F., Kathleen Grimes, Dana Davis, et al. "Clinical Precursors of Schizophrenia: Facial Expressions of Emotion." *American Journal of Psychiatry* 150 (1993): pp. 1655–60.

Walker, Elaine F., Tammy Savoie, and Dana Davis. "Neuromotor Precursors of Schizophrenia." *Schizophrenia Bulletin* 20 (1994): pp. 441–51.

Walker, John R. *Orphans of the Storm: Peacebuilding for Children of War.* Between the Lines, 1993.

Warrick, Pamela. "The Sad Truth About Men." *Los Angeles Times,* February 10, 1997, p. E1.

Watson, Traci. "Quieting the Voices: Schizophrenia Slowly Yields to New Treatments and New Understanding." *U.S. News and World Report,* October 28, 1996, p. 58.

Waxman, Laura. *A Status Report on Hunger and the Homeless in America's Cities: 1995.* Washington, D.C.: U.S. Conference of Mayors, 1995.

Weinberger, Daniel R. "From Neuropathology to Neurodevelopment." *The Lancet* 346 (1995): 552–57.

Werner, Emily E. "Resilient Children." In *Contemporary Readings in Child Psychology,* E. M. Hetherington and R. D. Parke, eds. New York: McGraw-Hill, 1987.

"Why Suicide Is Increasing Among Young Black Men." *JET,* August 1996, pp. 12–15.

Wingerson, Dane. "Awakenings—To What?" *The Journal of the California Alliance of the Mentally Ill* 7 (July 1996): pp. 12–14.

Woo, Elaine. "Prison Spending Hurts Schools and Black Students, Report Says." *Los Angeles Times,* October 23, 1996.

Wood, David. "The Children of War." *Atlanta Journal-Constitution,* March 31, 1996.

Woolis, Rebecca. *When Someone You Love Has a Mental Illness: A Handbook for Family, Friends, and Caregivers.* Los Angeles: J. P. Tarcher, 1991.

Wyatt, Richard Jed, and Ioline D. Henter. "Schizophrenia: An Introduction." *Brain Work: The Neuroscience Newsletter,* May/June 1997, p. 1.

Young, Mary Eming. *Early Child Development: Investing in the Future.* Washington, D.C.: The World Bank, 1996.

Index

Index